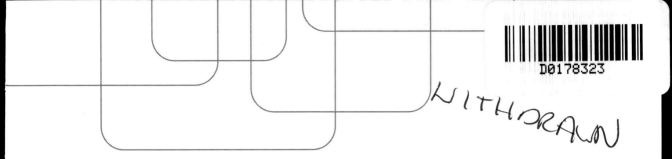

STUDY GUIDE
for OCR Psychology: A2 Level

LIN
150
GL

Fiona Lintern, Merv Stapleton & Lynne Williams

Hodder Arnold

A MEMBER OF THE HODDER HEADLINE GROUP

Orders: please contact Bookpoint Ltd, 130 Milton Park, Abingdon, Oxon OX14 4SB.
Telephone: +44 (0)1235 827720. Fax: +44 (0)1235 400454. Lines are open from 9.00–5.00,
Monday to Saturday, with a 24-hour message-answering service. You can also order through our website
www.hoddereducation.co.uk.

British Library Cataloguing in Publication Data
A catalogue record for this title is available from the British Library

ISBN-10: 0 340 81626 0
ISBN-13: 978 0 340 81626 4

First published 2004
Impression number   10 9 8 7 6 5 4 3
Year   2007 2006

Typeset by Dorchester Typesetting Group Ltd.
Printed in Great Britain for Hodder Arnold, an imprint of Hodder Education, a member of the Hodder Headline Group,
338 Euston Road, London NW1 3BH by Martins the Printers, Berwick-upon-Tweed.

Hodder Headline's policy is to use papers that are natural, renewable and recyclable products and made from wood
grown in sustainable forests. The logging and manufacturing process is expected to conform to the environmental
regulations of the country of origin.

CONTENTS

Contents

INTRODUCTION

The aim of this book

Students of OCR A2 Psychology have to study two out of six areas of applied psychology. These are:

1) psychology applied to education
2) psychology applied to health
3) psychology applied to organizations
4) psychology applied to environment
5) psychology applied to sport
6) psychology applied to crime.

These areas of psychology are covered in the *Psychology in Practice* series published by Hodder & Stoughton. These books address the eight areas required by the examination and include theoretical approaches and research, as well as activities designed to help you evaluate the material. This book is designed to complement that series. It is *not* a textbook and should be used alongside the textbook recommended by your teacher.

Recently, both students and teachers of the OCR specification have commented that more detail about a small number of pieces of research would be useful. Having details such as the sample, the forms of measurement used and other aspects of research should not only make it easier to understand the research but also simplify the identification of possible evaluation issues. This was the starting point for this book. We have identified a range of research evidence for each area of the specification and have summarized these studies for you.

We have taken outrageous liberties with some of the research, giving you a highly simplified version. We have broken down the aim of the research, often reporting only part of a longer study and focusing on key variables and measurements, a few important results and so on. In doing this, inevitably we have lost much of the depth and detail of the original articles. We hope the authors will forgive us.

We have also included an evaluation section after each set of research summaries. These are meant to give you an idea of how to evaluate and are not meant to be an exhaustive set of evaluation issues for each topic. You are strongly encouraged to develop your own set of evaluation issues for the examination. The rest of this introduction will show you how to evaluate and will explain exactly what the examiners are looking for.

How to evaluate psychological evidence

The first thing to realize is that evaluation is not difficult. Unfortunately, many students fail to gain marks in this section of the examination as they are not quite sure what they should be doing. As you read the evidence described in this book, think about what you are reading. Try to identify some issues that arise from the evidence which you think you would be able to discuss. These issues might be related to the way in which the research was conducted, the applications that might arise from the research or the theoretical perspectives on which the research is based.

It is virtually impossible to produce a complete list of evaluation issues, but the list provided below should point you in the right direction. Remember that different issues will feature more prominently in certain units and you should not worry if you cannot see the relevance of all of the following issues to the areas of applied psychology that you are studying.

Suggestions for evaluation issues

Research methods

There are many different issues that might be identified here. You could start with the following:

1) the strengths and weaknesses of the method used (experimental, observational etc.)
2) the strengths and weaknesses of the sample and sampling method (size, bias, is the sample representative of a larger population, would there be problems in generalizing from the sample?)
3) the ecological validity of the research (to what extent does the research reflect real life?)
4) the type of data that has been collected (e.g. you could discuss the strengths and weaknesses of qualitative and quantitative data)
5) the way that the variables have been controlled/manipulated/measured (what advantages/disadvantages can you identify?) – you could also consider any problems that might be associated with measuring complex variables, such as whether punishments or treatments reduce re-offending behaviours, whether people have job satisfaction or how environmental factors affect behaviour (this might overlap with the issue of reductionism)
6) the reliability and validity of the measurement
7) alternative explanations for the findings (can the results be explained in any other way or are there extraneous variables that have not been controlled?)
8) any other biases that can be identified in the research methodology (demand characteristics, social desirability bias, observer/experimenter bias etc.)
9) any ethical issues/implications arising from the research.

Theoretical/philosophical perspectives

There are a number of different theoretical perspectives in psychology (most importantly, you should be aware of cognitive, behaviourist, social, developmental, individual differences and physiological perspectives) that can be discussed. There are also some important philosophical debates that can be considered. These have more application to certain areas of applied psychology than others and you should not worry if you are unable to see the relevance of all of them. Try thinking about the following:

1) Which theoretical perspective is the evidence based upon? Are you able to compare evidence from two different theoretical perspectives (behaviourist versus cognitive approaches to education, for example, or social versus physiological explanations for criminal behaviour)? Does the evidence offer any support for a particular theoretical perspective?
2) Does the evidence aid our understanding of the nature/nurture debate or does it offer support for one side of this debate rather than the other? Comparisons between different pieces of evidence result in excellent evaluation.

3) Does the evidence tell us anything about the relative contributions of personality and situation to the explanation of behaviour? Compare if possible.
4) Does the evidence add to our understanding of the free will/determinism debate?
5) Is the evidence reductionist (reducing complex variables to simpler units)? What advantages and disadvantages does this have in relation to the aims of the research?
6) Does the evidence concentrate on one culture or does it compare different cultures? Could the research findings be generalized across cultures? Is there any evidence of ethnocentrism that could be discussed?
7) Have individual differences (these might be age differences, gender differences, cultural or social/demographic differences, occupational differences and so on) been considered?

Applications and implications

It is also worth considering the uses to which the evidence might be put. The following questions could be considered:
1) What practical applications might be suggested by the evidence? Is it clear how the evidence might be applied to real-life situations? This is obviously a particularly important issue in applied psychology. You could also consider any factors which prevent the evidence from being applied easily. This might include methodological problems, identified above.
2) How useful is the evidence? This obviously overlaps with the question about practical applications, but evidence is also useful if it advances our understanding of an issue. Evidence that identifies significant variables for further research or highlights important individual differences could also be considered useful. Take into account the methodological issues already identified when considering the issue of usefulness. Can research be useful if it has low ecological validity or if the sample is not representative?
3) Are there any ethical implications raised by the evidence? For example, some evidence might point to significant changes in practice, perhaps a change in educational policy, organizational work conditions or the potential treatment of patients or offenders. Have the ethical implications been explored fully? How might such changes affect individuals or groups?

The A2 examination

Each of the six units is examined in exactly the same way. You will sit an examination lasting $1\frac{1}{2}$ hours for each unit and these examinations are available in both January and June. Each paper has two sections and within each section there is a choice of two questions.

How to answer the examination questions

Section A (16 marks) – you will have a choice of one question from two in this section. You should spend approximately 30 minutes on this question.

Part a (6 marks) – this part of the question will always ask you to describe. You might be asked to describe a theory, an approach or some evidence. You should spend around ten minutes doing this, so you will be able to give a reasonable amount of detail. The examiners are looking for accurate information and evidence of understanding. Do not evaluate in part a – you will not get any marks for it.

Part b (10 marks) – this part of the question will always ask you to evaluate. This is likely to be more general than simply asking you to evaluate a single piece of research. For example, you might be asked to evaluate an approach or an issue (such as the advantages and disadvantages of using a particular method to investigate a particular topic). You must plan and structure the answer you give. It is better to select a few important issues to discuss in depth rather than simply producing a list of evaluation points. You have around 20 minutes to answer this part of the question, so you have time to fully explain your answer.

Section B (34 marks) – you will have a choice of one question from two in this section. You should spend approximately one hour on this question.

Part a (10 marks) – this question will always ask you to describe, but the focus of the question will be broader than in Section A. You should spend 15–20 minutes on this part of the question and aim to describe three or four pieces of evidence. The examiners are looking for accurate descriptions of evidence, use of psychological terms and concepts and evidence of understanding. The last is easy to achieve if you remember to explain the conclusions that can be drawn from each piece of evidence once you have described it. You could start a sentence with 'This evidence shows us that . . .'

Part b (16 marks) – this part of the question will always ask you to evaluate whatever you have just described in part a. There are more marks for this part of the question than for any other question on the paper, so you must make sure that you can do this (see above for suggested evaluation issues). You should spend 25–30 minutes on this part of the question. One of the best ways to answer this section is to select three (or more) evaluation issues that apply to the evidence you have described. You can then write about each evaluation in turn, relating this to as much of the evidence as you can. For example, you might write a paragraph on the strengths and weaknesses of the methods used, a paragraph on the ethics of the research, a paragraph on the samples and sampling methods and a paragraph on the usefulness of the research. The examiners are looking for evidence that you have identified and explained a number of relevant evaluation issues, related these issues clearly to the evidence, compared and contrasted the evidence wherever possible and demonstrated the ability to structure an argument. As with previous sections, ensure that you use psychological terms and concepts appropriately and that you explain your answer fully.

Part c (8 marks) – this part of the question will always ask you to apply psychological evidence to a real-life problem or situation. You should spend about 15 minutes on this part of the question and ensure that you support your suggestions with reference to psychological evidence. Once again, use of psychological terms and concepts and clarity of explanation will attract marks.

Section 1
EDUCATION

EDUCATION
Assessing educational performance

STUDY 1
Valencia, S. W., 1997, 'Authentic classroom assessment of early reading: alternatives to standardized tests', *Preventing School Failure*, 41, 2, 63–4

Aim

To provide evidence that standardized tests are not the only method of measuring reading ability in pupils in early years.

Method

A report of three case studies.

Participants

'Rebecca', a first-grade pupil, 'Laura', a fifth-grade student with special educational needs and 'Elizabeth', a third-grade student who had been assessed in every grade, from grades 1 to 3. All were pupils at a primary school in the USA.

Procedure

Authentic classroom assessment of early reading involves using activities that are similar to the everyday activities used in reading: students interact with real books, engage in meaningful discussion about them, write about what they have read and set their own goals. These activities involve the application of strategies and skills in many different reading contexts, as opposed to the isolated testing of such skills that is carried out via standardized assessment. Students are observed in a number of reading situations and the teacher is able to compile a profile of the reading skills and strategies they display and place them in context (i.e. which skills and strategies they use in which situation).

Rebecca had not yet started to read and so was tested for emergent reading skills, including such items as knowing the right way up for a book, knowing that books are read from left to right and front to back, being able to differentiate between letter, word and sentence and understanding the sequence of a story (beginning, middle and end). Three books suitable for emergent readers were placed in front of Rebecca and she was asked to pick one to read with the researcher. Her initial behaviour with the book was observed and recorded. As the researcher read the book with Rebecca, the latter was asked questions to elicit whether or not she understood what was happening in the story and what the pictures in the book showed. She was also encouraged to 'read' predictable, repetitive passages, along with the researcher. Rebecca was assessed on three different occasions.

Laura was tested for both emergent and beginning reading skills. The difference between these skill sets is, essentially, the ability to identify letters, words and sentences. Laura was asked to read aloud and observations of her reading behaviours were made.

Elizabeth was tested at least three times a year for three years on a range of reading behaviours; the books she was tested on ranged from easy to difficult for her age group. She was asked to read alone and to write down or draw pictures to represent what she had read; she also engaged in shared reading and questioning sessions with her teacher and with fellow pupils. A standardized form was used on all occasions to record the data about her reading ability. Elizabeth was also asked to self-evaluate her reading ability.

Case study 1 – Rebecca knew how to orient a book, move through it sequentially and use pictures to predict what was happening in the story. She was unable to read the print, but questioning revealed that she understood that print is read from left to right and from the top to the bottom of the page, the title of the book is found on the front cover and print, rather than pictures, is used to convey the story. She was unable, however, to identify letters, words and sentences.

Case study 2 – Laura showed the same range of emergent reading skills as Rebecca, but also was able to identify some letters and words. She was able to read aloud to a certain degree, but often used pictures rather than text to tell the story. Additionally, she often skipped words she found difficult, suggesting that she had not yet developed such strategies as using phonics to deal with unknown words. Laura also substituted words, this substitution being related to difficulties with recognizing vowels and word endings (e.g. she substituted 'worm' for 'warm' and 'looked' for 'learned'), and this hindered her ability to retell the story after reading it. When she was reading a story, however, she was able to retell it with little difficulty. This suggests that she was not reading for meaning, rather than lacking the ability to understand story structure.

Case study 3 – By the end of the first year, Elizabeth had high levels of listening comprehension, was able to summarize accurately many incidents from a story and her self-evaluation of her reading ability matched that of her teachers. By the end of the year she was able to read appropriately targeted books entirely on her own. By the end of the second year, Elizabeth was able to read age-appropriate books alone, self-correct her reading errors and read with expression.

STUDY 2

Cirino, P. T., Rashid, F. L., Sevcik, R. A., Lovett, M. W., Frijters, J. C., Wolf, M., Morris, R. D., 2002, 'Psychometric stability of nationally normed and experimental decoding and related measures in children with reading disability', *Journal of Learning Disabilities*, 35, 6, 525–39

Aim

To investigate the reliability of some nationally normed psychometric tests and other measures of reading for children with identified reading disabilities.

Method

Correlation.

Participants

78 children, aged 6.5–8.5 years, from schools in Atlanta, GA and Boston, MA in the USA and Toronto in Canada, who had been identified by their teachers as having reading disabilities. None of them had repeated a year at school and none had any major psychological disorders. 30 per cent of the sample was female, 17 per cent was left-handed and 49 per cent was black. 42 per cent of the children came from households that were classed as below average in socio-economic terms. All the participants spoke English as their first language and all had normal hearing and sight.

Procedure

All children identified by their teachers were given a screening battery of three tests:
1) the Kaufmann Brief Intelligence Test (K-BIT)
2) the Woodcock Reading Mastery Test – revised (WRMT-R)
3) the Wide Range Achievement Test – 3rd edition (WRAT-3).
The first test measures cognitive ability and the second and third measure reading ability. Only those scoring above 70 on the K-BIT but below average on the WRMT-R and WRAT-3 were included in the study.

Following the initial screening, over the following three months (April–June) the children were given the following tests:
1) Rapid Automatized Naming (RAN) and Rapid Alternating Stimuli (RAS) tests – to measure their speed and accuracy at naming objects, numbers, letters and letter–number combinations
2) Word Reading Efficiency sub-test of the Comprehensive Test of Reading Related Phonological Processes – to test ability to read words of increasing difficulty
3) Peabody Individual Achievement Test-Revised (PIAT-R) – to measure their ability to distinguish letters based on their sound, name and shape.
All the above tests have been normed for use on US schoolchildren of a similar age range to the participants.

In addition to these psychometric tests, the researchers devised some additional experimental measures of decoding, spelling and reading-related cognitive processes, primarily because none of the above tests had been developed for use with students with reading disabilities. These included three computer-administered, timed, word identification tests to measure the extent of automaticity of word identification, a test to measure learning transfer (the Challenge Test), a spelling test, a homophone/pseudohomophone test to assess correct word recognition based on sound and a test to assess their ability to combine phonemes into words.

All the above tests were re-administered in September and October of the same year and correlations between the two sets of scores were calculated as measures of test/re-test reliability. Differences between the two sets of scores were also analysed.

<table>
<tr><td>Results</td></tr>
</table>

Using the criterion of a correlation coefficient of 0.80 or above as indicating excellent test/re-test reliability, coefficients of 0.60–0.79 to indicate good test/re-test reliability and those below 0.60 as weak test/re-test reliability, the researchers found that all the nationally normed tests had good or excellent reliability for this group of participants, with the mean and median coefficients being 0.82.

The majority of the experimental measures were also found to have excellent or good test/re-test reliability (mean coefficient = 0.69, median = 0.68), but some of these measures (e.g. the spelling test and the Challenge Test of learning transfer) had only weak reliability. Further investigation of these variables revealed that they were not normally distributed, and when this was taken into consideration their reliability improved.

It was also found that there were strong correlations between scores on the nationally normed tests and their experimental equivalents. This suggests that the experimental measures used have concurrent validity.

Differences between the scores obtained in the April–June testing period and the September–October period across all measures were only very small, suggesting that improvements in reading for those with a reading disability are not simply a result of the passage of time.

STUDY 3
Nation, K., Clarke, P., Snowling, M. J., 2002, 'General cognitive ability in children with reading comprehension difficulties', *British Journal of Educational Psychology*, 72, 549–60

Aim
To investigate the cognitive abilities of children with reading comprehension difficulties.

Method
A quasi-experiment.

Participants
236 children in years 3 and 4 (aged 7–9 years) in a junior school in York were tested for their reading accuracy and reading comprehension, using the second version of the Neale Analysis of Reading Ability (NARA-II). Accuracy is measured by counting the number of words correctly read out loud and reading comprehension by their answers to questions about what they have just read. Additionally, decoding ability was assessed using the Graded Non-word Reading Test, in which the children read aloud non-words such as 'strumbesh' and 'tralishent'.

From this group, a sample of 25 children with reading comprehension difficulties were selected and matched on chronological age and word reading accuracy with 24 children with no reading comprehension difficulties. This is an imposed opportunity sample.

Procedure
The participants were given all six of the core scales of the British Ability Scales (2nd edition) School Age Battery (BAS-II); two of the scales measure verbal ability, two measure non-verbal ability and two measure spatial ability. Together they provide a measure of General Conceptual Ability (GCA). Additionally, combining scores from just the latter four scales provides a Special Non-Verbal Composite score. The children also underwent testing using a Word Reading and a Number Skills achievement test from the BAS-II.

The children were tested individually over two sessions of 30–45 minutes.

Results
Although both groups scored within the normal range of the BAS-II for GCA, those with reading comprehension difficulties scored significantly lower than those with no reading comprehension difficulties. In relation to the individual scales of the BAS-II, the greatest difference between the two groups lay in verbal ability, with those with reading comprehension difficulties scoring significantly lower than the control group. A similar, but not so great, difference was also found on the non-verbal scales. There were no significant differences in their spatial ability. The children with reading comprehension difficulties also scored significantly lower on the Special Non-Verbal Composite scale, thus suggesting that both verbal and non-verbal factors are implicated in the development of reading comprehension.

STUDY 4

Hatcher, J., Snowling, M. J., Griffiths, Y. M., 2002, 'Cognitive assessment of dyslexic students in higher education', *British Journal of Educational Psychology*, 72, 119–33

Aim

To investigate whether or not students with dyslexia have different cognitive skills to students who do not have dyslexia. A second aim was to assess the impact of cognitive difficulties on study skills.

Method

A quasi-experiment.

Participants

23 students with dyslexia and 50 control students were paid a small sum for volunteering to take part in the study. They were all undergraduate or postgraduate students at York University and were studying subjects across the entire academic range. The experimental group comprised 11 males and 12 females, aged 19–53 years (mean = 24 years 11 months), and the control group contained 16 males and 34 females, aged 18–41 years (mean = 21 years 8 months). Informed consent was obtained.

Procedure

The students underwent a battery of tests in a single session of 1.5–2 hours. The tests were followed by a number of counterbalanced writing, reading and fluency tasks, which are all aspects of study skills. The tests and tasks and what they were used to measure are shown in the table below.

Test	Variables measured
Wechsler Adult Intelligence Scale – revised (WAIS-R)	Verbal cognitive ability, speed of cognitive processing, verbal short-term memory
Raven's Advanced Progressive Matrices (short form)	Non-verbal cognitive ability
Wide Range Achievement Test – III Reading (blue and tan forms)	Reading, spelling
Brown Attention Deficit Disorder Scales (Brown ADD Scales)	Self-perception of attention and organizational skills
Nonsense passage reading	Decoding
Spoonerisms and rapid naming	Phonological skills
Graded difficulty arithmetic test	Mental arithmetic ability
Fluency tasks	Semantic, phonemic and rhyme fluency
Writing tasks	Writing speed, précis ability
Proofreading task	Ability to identify/misidentify errors in spelling, punctuation and grammar

| Results |

The group of students with dyslexia scored significantly lower on all tests of reading, spelling, cognitive processing, memory, phonological skills, mental arithmetic and fluency than the control group. Additionally, they took longer in the writing tasks and were less able to identify errors in the proofreading task. There was no significant difference in the IQ scores of the two groups as measured by the WAIS-R.

In relation to the writing, reading and fluency tasks, once again the students with dyslexia performed significantly worse than the control group.

The control group scored a mean of 60 on the Brown ADD Scales questionnaire, compared with a mean of 72 for the students with dyslexia, which was a significant difference. The higher the score, the more likely the diagnosis of ADD. Interestingly, the clinical cut-off point (i.e. the minimum score on the scale) for the likelihood of such a diagnosis is a score of 55 and both groups were above this score.

Evaluating research into assessing educational performance

Reliability, validity and standardization

One of the most important aspects of assessment of educational performance is that it should be reliable and valid, otherwise the assessment isn't worth the paper it is written on. Reliability is concerned with the consistency of a test. Of the studies outlined above, three use tests that are known to be reliable and valid for a normally distributed population, in other words, they are standardized tests. The Cirino *et al.* study also shows that the Kaufmann Brief Intelligence Test (K-BIT), the Woodcock Reading Mastery Test – revised (WRMT-R) and the Wide Range Achievement Test – 3rd edition (WRAT-3) also have test/re-test reliability for children with reading difficulties, and thus implies that they can be standardized for this population as well. The Hatcher *et al.* study, however, suggests that the same cannot be claimed for the Brown ADD Scales for university students. The fact that both the control and experimental groups scored higher than the clinical cut-off point for ADD diagnosis suggests that, for this group at least, this cut-off point is too low.

Ecological validity

For any conclusions from psychological research to have any real relevance, it is important that the research is conducted in such a way as to be close to the everyday experiences of its participants. This is a great strength of the authentic classroom assessment of reading approach taken in Valencia's case studies. The reading tasks given to the children and observed and recorded by their teacher were identical to the sort of reading tasks they would undertake during a normal schoolday. This cannot be said of the standardized reading tasks used in the Hatcher *et al.* and Nation *et al.* studies, where the reading tasks were taken out of context. It is not a part of everyday reading practice that we read lists of words or, indeed, nonsense words.

Methodology

The method used to conduct research has implications for the conclusions we can draw from it. While the case studies conducted by Valencia tell us in great detail about the effectiveness of authentic classroom assessment of reading on three individuals, we have to be careful about drawing any firm conclusions about how reliable and valid this approach would be when used on a wider sample. The correlation used in the Cirino *et al.* study, while appropriate for the purposes of the study – establishing the reliability of nationally normed tests for children with reading difficulties – tells us nothing about what causes those reading difficulties. The experimental methods used in the studies by Hatcher *et al.* and Nation *et al.*, however, do allow us to draw inferences about cause and effect. In the former, for example, it is possible to conclude that lowered verbal and non-verbal cognitive abilities are implicated in the development of reading comprehension difficulties, while in the latter we can conclude that dyslexia is not related to IQ, but can cause difficulties with developing sound study skills which, in turn, impact on educational achievement.

Usefulness

Given the emphasis on assessment in education, perhaps the most important use of the above studies is in revealing which assessments are appropriate for use with different students. Continuing to use the Brown ADD Scales with university students, for example, could result in many of them being misdiagnosed with ADD. Although this is highly unlikely, given that they are unlikely to be showing any of the symptoms of this disorder, this study does indicate that continuing to use this particular form of assessment for this group is problematical. The Cirino *et al.* study, on the other hand, tells us that the measures used in their study can be extended for use on children with reading difficulties. This means that educational psychologists have an additional tool to assist them in accurately identifying those with such difficulties. The same can be said for the use of the BAS-II, as used in the Nation *et al.* study.

EDUCATION
Design and layout of educational environments

STUDY 5
Gavienas, E., 'The dilemma: seating arrangements for group teaching', http://www.scre.ac.uk/rie/nl61/nl61gavienas.html (accessed 14 May 2004)

| Aim | To investigate whether the way group work sessions were organized affected the type of follow-up activity students were given to do while the teacher worked with other groups. |

Aim

To investigate whether the way group work sessions were organized affected the type of follow-up activity students were given to do while the teacher worked with other groups.

Method

Observation.

Participants

11 classes in a primary school.

Procedure

Prior to the observation the teachers were asked which curriculum areas they used group work for and all responded with maths and English, so these were the classes that were observed.

The researcher noted whether children were seated in social groups or ability groups and whether the teacher worked with these pre-formed groups at their table (visited them) or if children were extracted from the groups to form a new group when working with the teacher.

The type of follow-up task – oral, practical or written – was identified, as was whether it was an individual/paired or group task.

Following the observation the teachers were interviewed and questioned about the observations that had been made.

Results

Seven of the teachers extracted children in order to work with them, three teachers visited the groups and one teacher used a combination of extraction and visiting.

53 of the 72 follow-up tasks that were given were written tasks. There was no significant difference in the number of written tasks given by visiting or extracting teachers, but the former gave five times as many practical tasks. 62 of the 72 were individual tasks and this finding supports the subsequent interviews which revealed that visitors had not arranged their classroom layout to facilitate collaborative work on follow-up tasks, but rather to facilitate their movement from one group to another. It was also reported that extractors who sat children in social groups did so to try to limit the amount of talking during follow-up tasks. Having a mixed ability group would have resulted in fewer opportunities for effective collaboration and the need for talking that accompanies it.

The interviews revealed that the visitors' prime focus in organizing the seating arrangements as they had was in order to make it easier to share resources and this may have facilitated the increased number of practical follow-up tasks they used.

This was enhanced if the children were seated in ability groups rather than social groups.

It was also noted that extractors had to use a separate area of the classroom (usually a carpeted floor space with no furniture) for practical work and this impeded the demonstration of the practical work and the engagement of the children with it.

STUDY 6

McCroskey, J. C., McVetta, R. W., 'Classroom seating arrangements: instructional communication theory versus student preferences',
http://www.jamescmccroskey.com/publications/82.htm (accessed 14 May 2004)

Aim

This study was designed to examine students' preferences for three types of seating arrangements in relation to two variables: whether the course was mandatory or optional and the students' desire to communicate (their communication apprehension – CA). In particular, it was hypothesized that:

1) students will prefer to be seated in rows for mandatory courses, but in horseshoe or cluster arrangements for optional courses
2) students with high CA will show a stronger preference for seating arrangements that restrict opportunities for interaction compared to students with low CA
3) students with high CA will express greater preference for seats that allow a low level of participation in the classroom.

Method

A quasi-experiment.

Participants

972 college students who were taking two basic courses in communication at the same time. One was a lecture-based course, with over 300 students in each lecture, and the other was an experience-based course, with a maximum of 25 students per group.

Procedure

All participants were required to complete the Personal Report of Communication Apprehension (PRCA), a 24-item inventory which measures feelings about communication with others using a 5-point Likert scale (1 = strongly agree, 5 = strongly disagree). It has been shown to have high internal reliability and predictive validity. In this study, those scoring one SD or more above the mean were classified as having high CA, while those one SD or more below the mean were classed as having low CA. Those between +/-1 SD were classed as moderate CA. The PRCA was completed during one of the experience-based course sessions.

To measure preferences for seating arrangements and whether or not they preferred high-, moderate- or low-interaction seat positions, the students were given diagrams similar to that shown below. They were asked to indicate which arrangement they generally preferred, which they preferred for a mandatory course that they did not want to take and which arrangement they preferred for an optional course. In addition, they were asked to mark with an 'x' which seat they would prefer to sit in for each arrangement. On the actual diagrams given to the students, the seats were numbered rather than being shaded as they are in the diagram below:

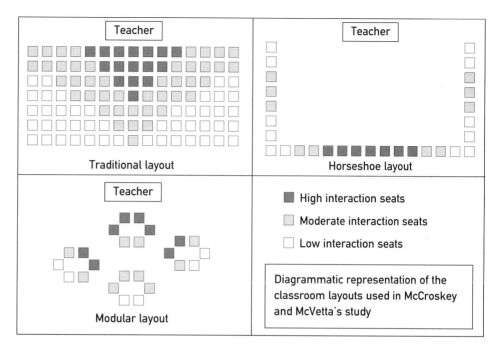

Diagrammatic representation of the classroom layouts used in McCroskey and McVetta's study

Once collected, the data were submitted to a chi-squared analysis.

The results are shown in the table below in terms of percentages that preferred each layout in general, for mandatory and optional courses:

Course	Traditional	Horseshoe	Modular
General preference	48%	34%	18%
Mandatory	55%	14%	31%
Optional	32%	44%	23%

Thus while there was a general preference for traditional seating arrangements for nearly half the sample, the type of course had a significant effect on seating arrangement preference.

In relation to communication apprehension, as a general preference, those with low CA favoured the horseshoe arrangement while those with moderate and high CA favoured the traditional layout.

All three groups expressed a preference for the traditional layout for mandatory courses and the strength of this preference was in line with the degree of CA they reported.

For optional courses all students expressed a preference for the horseshoe arrangement, with low CA students expressing the strongest preference.

With regard to preference for low-, moderate- or high-interaction seating places, as predicted, students with high CA expressed a greater preference for low-interaction seats than they did for moderate- or high-interaction seats. Similarly, those with low CA preferred high-interaction seats.

STUDY 7
Merrett, F., Wheldall, K., 1990, *Positive Teaching in the Primary School*, London: Paul Chapman Publishers

Aim	To investigate the effects of seating arrangements in top junior classes on students' on-task behaviour.
Method	Experiment with repeated measures design.
Participants	A class of 28 boys and girls in a junior school in an urban residential area and a second class of 25 boys and girls in a school on a council housing estate. All the children were aged 10–11 years and were in mixed ability classes.
Procedure	In both classes the usual seating arrangement was around tables in groups and the children were observed for a two-week period in this setting. An observation schedule was drawn up and used to measure the amount of on-task behaviour exhibited. On-task behaviour was defined as the children doing what the teachers asked of them e.g. paying attention when they were talking, reading books and work-cards when given tasks to do and only being out of their seat with permission.

Following this two-week period of observation, and without commenting on it to the children, the teachers rearranged the seating into rows. The children's on-task behaviour was again observed for a second two-week period before the original seating arrangement was reinstated (again without comment from the teachers) and they were observed for a further two weeks.

Results	In both classes on-task behaviour increased by approximately 15 per cent when they were seated in rows, and fell by almost the same amount when they returned to group seating. The largest improvements (over 30 per cent) were shown by those whose initial amount of on-task behaviour had been lowest. There was a much less marked effect for those whose initial on-task behaviour had been high.

It was also noted that, on the return to the group seating arrangement, children in both classes complained about the change, thus indicating a preference for seating in rows.

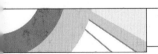

Evaluating research into design and layout of educational environments

Ecological validity
The importance of ecological validity in relation to research into the design and layout of educational environments should be obvious. How can we know for certain the effects of layout and design on academic-related behaviour and performance if the research is not conducted in real classrooms with real students? This is precisely what was done by Gavienas and Merrett and Wheldall in their studies and this means that we can have a high degree of confidence in their findings. The McCroskey and McVetta study, however, is lower in ecological validity than the

other two as, although real students were used, the use of diagrams to indicate seating preferences rather than in vivo interviews and observations means that there is more room for error. For example, some students in this study may have mistakenly put a cross in a high-interaction seat that was next to a moderate-interaction seat that they had intended to choose.

Determinism and free will

Determinism is the concept that all human behaviour has an identifiable cause which, to all intents and purposes, is beyond our control rather than the result of our exercising choice or free will. One form of determinism is environmental determinism, where the cause for behaviour lies in the surrounding environment. In the Merrett and Wheldall study the change in student behaviour, as far as the researchers are concerned, is a direct result of manipulating the environment, and Gavienas reported that the teachers elected to lay out their classroom furniture in order to control the behaviour of their students, so both studies support the concept of environmental determinism. The McCroskey and McVetta study, however, is more difficult to place in relation to the determinism debate. In examining the association between seating arrangements and type of course, for example, it is difficult to say whether the seating arrangements affect the choice of courses taken or the other way round. If it is the former, then environmental determinism is at work; if the latter, is this free will or coincidence?

Generalization

Of the studies described above, two (those of Gavienas and Merrett and Wheldall) were carried out in primary schools, so we should be cautious about extending their findings to other educational settings. Do teachers in secondary and further education, for example, have as much control over the layout and design of their classrooms as the teachers in the Gavienas study, given that many classrooms are a shared resource in such institutions? Would older students respond in the same way as the primary school students to changes in their seating arrangements, as shown by Merrett and Wheldall? If we cannot be certain about this, we have to be careful about over-generalizing.

Usefulness

All these studies provide food for thought for teachers when it comes to considering the design and layout of their classrooms. The Gavienas study, for instance, suggests that the classroom layout can be used to control the amount of off-task behaviour by arranging seating in groups and populating those groups with children of mixed rather than similar ability. The Merrett and Wheldall study, on the other hand, implies that teachers can increase the amount of on-task behaviour by seating students in rows, although it tells us nothing about the quality of the work undertaken in rows compared to groups. The McCroskey and McVetta study carries with it the implication that a possible factor for teachers to consider when arranging their classroom furniture is the popularity of the course, as it would seem that whether or not students like a course affects their seating arrangement preference.

EDUCATION
Disruptive behaviour

STUDY 8

Handen, B. L., McAuliffe, S., Janosky, J., Feldman, H., Breaux, A. M., 1994, 'Classroom behaviour and children with mental retardation: comparison of children with and without ADHD', *Journal of Abnormal Child Psychology*, 22, 3, 267–81

Aim

To investigate whether or not children with low IQ scores and diagnosed as having ADHD exhibit more disruptive behaviour in the classroom than children with low IQ scores but without ADHD.

Method

A quasi-experiment.

Participants

The sample consisted of 34 children, aged 6–12 years (mean = 9.4 years), with an IQ score of 50–77 (mean = 65). 17 of the children had been diagnosed with ADHD previously, via a semi-structured DSM-III-R interview, and all scored 15+ on the Hyperactivity Index of both the Conners Teacher Rating Scale (administered by their schoolteacher) and Conners Parent Rating Scale (administered by their parents). These participants formed the experimental group. 59 per cent of this group were male and 77 per cent were white. The remaining 17 children, who all scored 11 or less on the two Conners Scales, formed the control condition. 53 per cent of this group were male and 88 per cent were white.

Procedure

All the subjects were participants in a Saturday laboratory school programme held at a hospital in Pittsburgh as part of a study into the effects of stimulants in controlling ADHD. Sessions lasted for six hours, from 9 a.m. to 3 p.m. During the first two Saturdays of the stimulants study, the children were drug-free to allow baseline measurements to take place. The data gathered during this period were used for this study on differences in disruptive behaviour.

During the Saturday school a 12-minute structured group activity was organized, with three to five participants in each group. This represented a simulation of a classroom group instruction session. The participants were individually observed once every 90 seconds for ten-second intervals during this session and their on-task, in-seat and fidgeting behaviours were recorded. Additionally, using a 5-point Likert scale, global ratings for restlessness and task interest were recorded at the end of the session for each child. Each child also had an actometer strapped to their ankle to measure the extent of their physical activity.

An individual 12-minute work task, involving a pencil and paper task covering recently mastered material was also given to groups of three to five participants. The measures taken and the method of recording the data was the same as for the group task. An additional measurement of the percentage of the tasks that were performed correctly was also taken.

In order to validate the ratings given to the children by their teachers and parents, the children were also rated on the Conners Teacher Rating Scale and the Child Attention Problems Behaviour Checklist (CAP). The former is a 28-point behaviour checklist with four sub-scales:

1) Conduct Problems
2) Hyperactivity
3) Inattention-Passivity
4) Hyperactivity Index.

Each item is rated on a 4-point scale for frequency of occurrence (0 = not at all, 3 = very much). The Hyperactivity Index is a 12-point behaviour checklist with three sub-scales:

1) Overactive
2) Inattentive
3) Total Score.

Each item is rated on a 3-point scale (0 = not true, 2 = very true). Additionally, inter-rater reliability testing was conducted on 20 per cent of the total observations recorded.

The Saturday school staff were blind to the study. They were also unaware of the existence of the control group, as the programme, as far as they were aware, was for children with low IQ and ADHD only.

| Results |

In relation to the group task, there was no significant difference between the control and experimental groups on any of the three measures (on-task, in-seat and fidgeting) taken. It should be noted, however, that the actometer readings were much higher for the ADHD group (112) than the control group (57) and approached significance ($p<.07$). Significant differences between the groups were found on the measures of global restlessness and task interest, with the ADHD group displaying more restlessness and less interest in the task than the control group.

In relation to the individual task, the ADHD group showed significantly lower on-task behaviour, more global restlessness and higher actometer readings. There was no significant difference in the percentage of individual tasks that the two groups performed correctly.

There was a significant positive correlation between the scores given by the teacher, parents and researchers on the Conners Scales and the CAP. Inter-rater reliability was found to be 99 per cent for in-seat behaviour, 92 per cent for on-task behaviour and 80 per cent for fidgeting.

STUDY 9

Abikoff, H. B., Jensen, P. S., Arnold, L. L. E., Hoza, B., Hechtman, L., Pollack, S., Martin, D., Alvir, J., March, J. S., Hinshaw, S., Vitiello, B., Newcorn, J., Greiner, A., Cantwell, D. P., Conners, C. K., Elliott, G., Greenhill, L. L., Kraemer, H., Pelham, W. E., Jr., Severe, J. B., Swanson, J. M., Wells, K., Wigal, T., 2002, 'Observed classroom behaviour of children with ADHD: relationship to gender and co-morbidity', *Journal of Abnormal Child Psychology*, 30, 4, 349–60

Aim

Generally the aim was to investigate gender and co-morbidity differences in the observed classroom behaviour of children with attention deficit hyperactivity disorder. The following specific hypotheses were tested:
1) children with ADHD will exhibit significantly more ADHD-associated behaviours than children without ADHD
2) boys with ADHD will exhibit significantly more rule-breaking and other externalizing behaviours than girls with ADHD
3) there will be no significant difference in the level of inattention and fidgeting shown by boys and girls with ADHD
4) children with ADHD and co-morbid anxiety (ANX) will be significantly less hyperactive, less impulsive and exhibit lower rates of rule-breaking than children with ADHD alone and those with ADHD and co-morbid Disruptive Behaviour Disorders (DBDs) – specifically Conduct Disorder (CD) and Oppositional Defiant Disorder (ODD)
5) children with co-morbid DBDs will exhibit significantly higher rates of rule-breaking, impulsive and aggressive behaviours than any other group.

Method

A quasi-experiment.

Participants

The experimental group comprised 403 boys and 99 girls, aged 7–10 years (mean = 8.4 years), all of whom had been diagnosed via a Diagnostic Interview Schedule for Children – Parent Report (DISC-P) with ADHD. Some children whose DISC-P reading indicated that they were just below the threshold for ADHD diagnosis were included if their teachers had observed up to two ADHD symptoms in their behaviour. Additionally, all had scores at least greater than one standard deviation above the mean on the Parents and Teachers Conners Scales. In addition, they all achieved a score in excess of 80 on the WISC-III Full Scale Verbal or Performance IQ or a similar score on the Scales for Independent Behaviour. 12 per cent of the experimental group had co-morbid anxiety, 34 per cent had co-morbid DBD, 22 per cent had both co-morbid anxiety and DBD and the remaining 32 per cent only had ADHD. A group of non-ADHD-diagnosed children, matched for age and ethnicity and from the same school class as the experimental group, acted as controls. 64 per cent of the sample was Caucasian, 19 per cent African-American, 6 per cent Hispanic and the remainder came from other ethnic groups.

Procedure

The participants were observed during normal teaching sessions using the Classroom Observation Code (COC). This observation schedule contains behavioural categories such as interference (e.g. talking during work, clowning about), interference to teacher (e.g. interrupting the teacher), off-task, non-compliance to teacher, physical and verbal aggression and so on. It is known to have construct validity. Observations were made in 15-second intervals over a period of four minutes for each participant and, for most categories, only the first occurrence of a behaviour was recorded. For three categories (off-task, out-of-chair and non-compliance) a timed criterion is required, so these were only scored if they occurred for the full 15-second interval.

All observers were trained using instruction, scoring of videos and scoring in real classrooms. Only those who achieved an inter-rater reliability in excess of 70 per cent on three consecutive classroom training sessions were used to collect data. Observers were informed prior to observation of the classroom rules utilized by the teacher in whose class they were to be observing. The observers were blind as to which condition the participants belonged. Additional inter-rater reliability for data gathered during the actual study was also calculated.

Results

Inter-rater reliability was found to be 80 per cent or greater. The following results were obtained:

1) the general hypothesis, that children with ADHD will exhibit significantly more ADHD-associated behaviours than children without ADHD, was supported
2) in relation to gender, the hypothesis that boys with ADHD will exhibit significantly more rule-breaking and other externalizing behaviours than girls with ADHD was also supported
3) the hypothesis that there will be no significant difference in the level of inattention and fidgeting shown by boys and girls with ADHD was supported
4) in relation to co-morbidity, the hypothesis that children with ADHD and co-morbid anxiety will be significantly less hyperactive, less impulsive and exhibit lower rates of rule-breaking than children with ADHD alone and those with ADHD and co-morbid Disruptive Behaviour Disorders (specifically Conduct Disorder and Oppositional Defiant Disorder), was rejected
5) the hypothesis that children with co-morbid DBDs will exhibit significantly higher rates of rule-breaking, impulsive and aggressive behaviours than any other group was supported.

STUDY 10
Van der Heyden, A. M., Witt, J, C., Gatti, S., 2001, 'Descriptive assessment method to reduce overall disruptive behaviour in a pre-school classroom', *School Psychology Review*, 30, 4, 548–68

Aim	This study had two main aims. The first was to develop a brief assessment tool that could be used in the classroom to identify naturally occurring, high-frequency events acting as reinforcers of disruptive behaviour. The second was to investigate whether or not the withholding of these reinforcers would result in lowered disruptive behaviour.

Method	A descriptive method to develop the tool and then an experiment to test the efficacy of the tool.

Participants	Two classrooms were used. Classroom 1 was in a pre-school centre for children with speech development delays. In this classroom were eight children, aged 2–4 years, a head teacher (with a Masters level degree in speech pathology), a graduate student of speech pathology and two classroom assistants. Three of the children had been diagnosed with autism and one with hypothyroidism.

In classroom 2, which was in a Head Start centre, there were 22 children, but, due to time considerations, six of these were selected at random to participate in this study.

Informed consent was obtained from the parents of all children in the study.

Procedure	Tool development – the teacher in each class was asked to identify which activity provided them with the greatest problem in terms of amount of disruptive behaviours. They both identified 'the circle activity', in which the children sit in a circle and a teacher-led activity, such as reading or singing, takes place. During this activity, the children were afforded multiple opportunities to respond (both verbally and non-verbally) and were expected to show turn-taking skills, stay in their seats and pay attention to the teacher. Two researchers were present during this session. One acted as an additional classroom assistant and interacted with the children as instructed by the teacher; the other acted as an observer. The children and teachers were observed individually in ten-second intervals. Two behaviours for target children, one peer behaviour and five to eight teacher behaviours were recorded. Behaviour categories used were attention, tangible, demand, compliance, escape and disruptive behaviour. The first five of these were recorded for their occurrence both just before (antecedent) and just after (subsequent) the occurrence of the disruptive behaviour on a tally chart. All observers were trained and inter-rater reliability was established as exceeding 90 per cent.

Following this, the teachers were informed of the outcomes and, in conjunction with the researchers, identified which behaviours acted as reinforcers for disruptive behaviours. It was found that attention from the teacher was the most significant behaviour that occurred subsequent to disruptive behaviour and, therefore, was likely to act as a reinforcer for that disruptive behaviour. Peer attention was the next most common factor.

Experimental testing – using a repeated measures design, the teachers were instructed either to attend to the children by rewarding them for their appropriate behaviour (e.g. by praising them) while ignoring their disruptive behaviour, or to give their attention to the children as a consequence of their disruptive behaviour by reprimanding them and ignoring any appropriate behaviours. Data from the tool development phase was used as baseline data for the experimental phase.

Results

The results from the tool development phase indicate that teacher attention is the single most important reinforcer of disruptive behaviour in the classroom.

Analysis of the data from the experimental phase showed that the total amount of teacher attention given in both the rewarding and reprimanding conditions was the same. This rules out the possibility that the amount of teacher attention was a confounding variable.

Disruptive behaviour occurred in 31 per cent of the observation intervals in the baseline sessions. In the reprimand sessions, it fell slightly to 27 per cent, but in the rewarding sessions it fell to 16 per cent.

> **STUDY 11**
> Breunlin, D. C., Cimmarusti, R. A., Bryant-Edwards, T. L., Hetherington, J. S., 2002, 'Conflict resolution training as an alternative to suspension for violent behaviour', *The Journal of Educational Research*, 95, 6, 349–59

Aim

To investigate whether or not conflict resolution training acts as an alternative to suspension from school for aggressive behaviour. In particular, four hypotheses were tested:
1) students who undertake conflict resolution training will have lower rates of re-suspension for physical violence than those who do not undertake such training
2) those who undertake such training will also have lower rates of re-suspension for verbal aggression
3) those students who follow this training will have a lower overall re-suspension rate
4) those who complete such a programme will have a reduced record of disciplinary actions taken against them than those who do not complete such a programme.

Method

Experiment, with a repeated measures design.

Participants

165 first- and second-year US high school pupils, who had been suspended from school between August 1997 and December 1998.

Procedure

At the start of the study, data on the discipline and suspension records of all the students in the school were gathered. Those who had been suspended were selected for inclusion in the study and their discipline and suspension records were utilized to provide baseline data. The number of incidents, the type of incident and the reasons for suspension/disciplinary action and so on were recorded.

The usual way of dealing with aggressive behaviour in the school was via suspension from school for a number of days, the length of suspension being related to the severity of the incident. From January 1999, assistant principals at the school, who were responsible for disciplinary procedures, agreed to refer students suspended for fighting and other aggressive acts to a conflict resolution training programme devised by the researchers. If the students agreed to attend they received a reduction in the number of days they were to be suspended from school. Failure to complete the programme resulted in the reinstatement of the original suspension length. Some students who were suspended for non-violent infringements of the school rules were also referred to the programme.

The training programme, labelled the Alternative to Suspension for Violent Behaviour (ASVB), included teaching the students the use of social problem-solving and thinking skills. The entire programme was grounded on previous psychological research into factors that reduce aggressive behaviours.

Results

For purposes of analysis, the participants were divided into six groups:
1) those suspended for fighting who undertook the programme (n = 25)
2) those suspended for fighting who did not attend the programme (n = 41)

3) those suspended for other aggressive behaviours who attended the programme (n = 7)
4) those suspended for other aggressive behaviours who did not attend the programme (n = 36)
5) those suspended for non-violent acts who attended the training (n = 10)
6) those suspended for non-violent acts who did not attend the training (n = 46).

It was found that, overall, students who undertook the ASVB conflict resolution training received fewer re-suspensions than those who did not. It was also found that there were no expulsions from among the former groups, while seven students who opted not to follow the programme were expelled for further aggressive behaviour. Students in group 1 were twice less likely than those in group 2, five times less likely than those in group 4 and four times less likely than those in group 6 to be re-suspended.

It was also found that the overall disciplinary records of those in group 1 improved significantly more than the records of those in group 2.

Evaluating research into disruptive behaviour

Ecological validity

If we are to be in a position to place faith in the conclusions drawn from psychological research, it is important that the data on which those conclusions are based is gathered in a way that bears more than a passing resemblance to the everyday lives of the participants in that research. In relation to research into disruptive behaviour at school, this means that the research should have been conducted in a real school setting, using tasks and procedures that were part of the everyday life of that school. This is certainly true of the Abikoff et al., Van der Heyden et al. and Breunlin et al. studies. All three studies took place in the participants' usual school lessons and were integrated into the daily school life of the students. It could be argued, however, that the Breunlin et al. study is somewhat lower in ecological validity than the other two as the conflict resolution programme was not part of the usual curriculum experienced by the students. Perhaps even lower in ecological validity is the Handen et al. study, in which a simulated classroom setting was used as part of the procedure. It may be that the behaviour of the participants in this study would have been different if the study had been conducted in the more familiar surroundings of their own school.

Reliability and validity

Almost inevitably, research into disruptive behaviour involves the collection of data by observation. In order to avoid the possibility of observations being subjective, it is important that agreed observational categories are drawn up and that the researchers' interpretation of those categories and their recording of behavioural occurrences against them are consistent. If they are not, we can have no confidence in the validity of the data and any conclusions drawn from them. It is generally accepted that a correlation of 70–75 per cent or greater between different observers' recordings is sufficient for inter-rater reliability to be established. Handen et al., with 80–99 per cent, Abikoff et al., with 80+ per cent, and Van der Heyden et al., with 90 per cent correlations between their respective observers, undoubtedly all established inter-rater reliability to acceptable standards.

Generalization

Generalization is the process of extending the conclusions drawn from the findings of a research study from the sample on which the research was conducted to the wider population from which that sample was drawn. There are a number of factors which limit the ability to generalize. One of the most important is sample size. Abikoff *et al.*'s sample of 502 participants presents no problem in this regard, and the same could be said of Breunlin *et al.*'s sample of 165 students who had been suspended from school. The Handen *et al.* study (34 participants) and the Van der Heyden *et al.* study (14 participants) have to be treated with more caution when it comes to generalizing, however. On the other hand, the Handen *et al.* study involved children with low IQ scores, a relatively small population, so it is almost inevitable that samples drawn from such a population will be small, and therefore generalizing to such a population from a smaller sample is more reasonable.

Usefulness

While investigating disruptive behaviour in order to develop knowledge and understanding of it may be worthwhile, it could be argued that the development of strategies and programmes to control or prevent such behaviour is even more important. Thus while the Handen *et al.* and Abikoff *et al.* studies increase our knowledge of our ability to identify accurately features of disruptive behaviour in particular groups of children, it could be argued that the conclusions of the Van der Heyden *et al.* and Breunlin *et al.* studies are far more useful. The former suggests that, via observation of their own and their students' behaviour, teachers can develop an understanding of the relationship between them and, via modifying their own behaviour, can bring about change in the disruptive behaviour of their students. The Breunlin *et al.* study's usefulness lies in the fact that it demonstrates that a carefully constructed programme of teaching, based on theory and research, can also modify the disruptive behaviour of school students.

EDUCATION
Individual differences in educational performance: cultural diversity and gender issues

---

STUDY 12
Mellanby, J., Martin, M., O'Doherty, J., 2000, 'The "gender gap" in final examination results at Oxford University', *British Journal of Psychology*, 91, 3, 377–94

Aim

To investigate whether or not gender differences in examination results at Oxford University are the consequence of individual differences between the genders.

Method

A quasi-experiment.

Participants

232 undergraduate students (117 female, 115 male) volunteered to take part in this study. They were recruited by three methods:
1) via tutors
2) by asking for volunteers at the end of a lecture (all students present having previously received a letter to inform them of the study)
3) by advertisement on noticeboards and mailshots targeted at specific course areas.
All volunteers were entered into a prize draw as an incentive to participate. The students were all in their final year and were studying chemistry (35), modern languages (28), biochemistry (23), modern history (22), physics (20), law (20), geography (21), biological sciences (19), English (18), classics (12), mathematics (ten) and engineering sciences (nine). They all had similar A level grades and were representative of Oxford undergraduates in terms of their previous academic achievements. Written consent was given by the students for their final examination mark to be used for the purposes of the study. Confidentiality of the data was guaranteed.

Procedure

The researchers constructed an extensive questionnaire by combining items from previously validated scales, modifying items from other scales and developing items especially for this study. The items on the questionnaire were designed to measure the following constructs:
1) ability/aptitude
2) motivation
3) mood
4) self-esteem/efficacy
5) interpersonal relationships
6) working patterns.
An initial pilot study was conducted on 65 final-year students to test out the validity and reliability of the questionnaire. As a consequence of this pilot, several items were removed from the questionnaire.

The questionnaire was conducted in a classroom setting, two to three months before the students' finals and took just under one hour to complete.

An average of the marks awarded for all final examinations sat by each participant was calculated.

The questionnaire responses for each of the six constructs listed above were analysed to see if there were any gender differences. The researchers also examined the ability of these constructs to predict examination results. Only those constructs in which there was a gender difference and which also reliably predicted examination results could be said to contribute to the gender gap.

Results

The female students scored slightly lower on the non-verbal items of the ability/aptitude test (and this was especially true of science students), but overall there was no significant difference between their scores and those of the male students. The verbal items were better predictors of examination marks than the non-verbal items.

The female students revealed a greater 'work ethic' than the male students, but overall there was no significant difference in their academic motivation. There was no relationship between scores on the motivation scale and examination marks.

The male students scored more highly on happiness and loneliness items than the female students, while the latter scored higher on depression and anxiety. For the males, loneliness was a weak predictor of examination success, while there was a surprising relationship between scores on the depression items and examination marks for the female students – the more depressed the better the marks.

Male students scored higher on self-esteem/efficacy items than females (e.g. used more high-risk revision methods, such as question-spotting), but there was no relationship with examination marks.

There were no gender differences in responses to items on interpersonal relationships.

In terms of working patterns, the female students worked independently for a longer time than the male students. Again, there was no relationship between scores on the working pattern scale and examination results.

In summary, although there are some gender differences in motivation, mood, self-esteem and working patterns, none of these factors has predictive validity for examination results.

The only construct with such predictive validity is verbal assessment of ability/aptitude, for which this study found no gender differences.

The authors conclude that the actual gender differences in terms of the ratio of different classes of degrees awarded to males and females (the former are awarded proportionally more first class degrees, for instance) is far more likely to be related to the nature of the academic assessment system than it is to individual differences between the genders.

STUDY 13

'Talk, gender and teachers' questioning in English lessons', http://www.standards.dfes.gov.uk/midbins/keystage3/cs_itt_gender.DOC (accessed 14 May 2004 – no details of author provided on the website)

Aim

To investigate whether the better educational performance of girls than boys at Key Stages 3 and 4 in English was a consequence of pupil/teacher behaviour and attitudes surrounding gender, talk and questioning.

Method

Case study utilizing observation, semi-structured interviews and teacher assessment of students' work to gather data.

Participants

Students and teachers in six English classes in a mixed comprehensive school in London.

Procedure

Observations and covert recordings of the classroom interactions were made and analysed, using Bloom's Taxonomy to identify whether teachers were asking more questions of boys than girls and also to identify the types of questions being asked. Covert recordings of small group work were also undertaken to gather data of peer interaction and semi-structured interviews were held with students to gather their views on classroom dynamics.

The observer also took notes recording the teachers' use of praise and concurrent non-verbal communications to provide data about how talk is conducted as well as what is said; and in order to assess covert gender bias, teachers were asked to assess whether the interviewee in a series of unattributed interview transcripts was a boy or a girl.

Results

Data from the observations revealed that boys were asked twice as many questions as girls and were asked four times as many open, explorative and analytical questions, requiring higher order thinking skills to answer them. It was also found that boys were five times more likely to interrupt other students' responses than girls were.

From the interviews it was discovered that seven out of the ten 'best speakers' identified by the students were boys, and girls were identified as those who spoke least in class. Additionally, all the students preferred working in single-sex groups.

In terms of covert gender bias, an analysis of the teachers' accreditation of the unattributed interview transcripts to boys or girls revealed that teachers associated filled pauses and hesitancy with girls rather than boys and believed that those who identified themselves as being lazy or disruptive were boys while girls perceived themselves as helpful and cooperative.

These findings suggest that the better achievement of girls in English at Key Stages 3 and 4 is not, in fact, contributed to by the gender discrepancies in talk that exist in the English classroom.

STUDY 14
Cline, T., de Abreu, G., Fihosy, C., Gray, H., Lambert, H., Neale, J., 2002, 'Minority ethnic pupils in mainly white schools', *Research Report* 365, DfES/HMSO

Aim	

One of the main aims of this multifaceted research was to investigate the academic achievement of minority ethnic students in predominantly white schools. This summary focuses primarily on this aspect of the research.

Method	

Survey and case studies.

Participants	

Over 34,000 students from schools from 35 different Local Education Authorities (LEAs) in England with 4–6 per cent minority ethnic students. From this sample, a sub-sample of students (from years 3–6 in primary and years 7–9 in secondary schools) from 14 schools from different areas of the country was selected to take part in a series of case studies. Additionally, parents and teachers of 61 ethnic minority students were also part of the sample.

Procedure	

First, data was gathered from the records of the LEAs of the Key Stage 2 and GCSE results for all pupils in the target schools.

During the case studies, the selected pupils, both white and ethnic minority, completed a questionnaire that was designed to gather data on their perceptions of school life and the support they received at home for their education.

This was then followed by a series of interviews with 61 ethnic minority students, their parents and a sample of 77 of their teachers to gain additional detail to support the findings of the survey.

Results	

The data on Key Stage 2 and GCSE results revealed that white pupils in mainly white schools achieved higher grades than white children in urban multi-ethnic schools. The same data also revealed that students from black Caribbean, Indian and Pakistani backgrounds outperformed their counterparts in urban multi-ethnic schools at GCSE level, but not at the end of Key Stage 2.

From the data gathered via the case studies and interviews, it was found that there was very little difference between students from ethnic minorities and white students in terms of their negative and positive perceptions of school and home support. There was a slight tendency for white students to give positive responses overall, but they were also more likely to reveal a negative perception on academic matters. The two items which minority ethnic students raised more than white students were the lack of support in preparing them for living in a multiracial society and bullying, particularly race-related name-calling and abuse.

It was also found that, while schools had strategies and practices in place to support students for whom English was not their first language in the initial stages of their time at school, none provided support beyond that period. The researcher also found that there were very few instances of attempts to incorporate cultural diversity into curriculum areas and that this was noted by the ethnic minority students, who felt a little undervalued as a result.

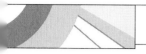

Evaluating research into individual differences in educational performance: cultural diversity and gender issues

Ethics

There are a number of ethical issues raised when conducting research into individual differences in educational performance. Probably the most important is that of confidentiality/anonymity. Any research into educational performance inevitably uses examination marks/grades as the dependent variable. It is very important that the research does not allow the names of any individuals who received particular grades to be published, unless, of course, the researchers have the prior consent of those involved. Anonymity/confidentiality was maintained in all these studies. Additionally, because of the fact that it may impact on teacher–student relationships, the study on talk, gender and teachers' questioning in English lessons involved the use of unattributed transcripts to prevent the teacher from identifying any individual.

Qualitative/quantitative data

One of the major strengths of quantitative data is that it can be used for statistical analysis and so lend scientific credibility to a study. For example, the use of numerical scales in the Mellanby *et al.* study and the percentage achievement rates provided by the LEAs in the Cline *et al.* study provide convincing arguments for the claims made by the respective researchers about the differing ability and educational performance/underperformance of the students in those studies. What such data do not tell us, however, are the reasons why such differences have occurred. This is why both these research studies utilized additional qualitative data. This type of data allows students to express in their own terms reasons for their educational performance.

Nature/nurture

There has been, and continues to be, an ongoing debate about whether or not differences in behaviour (including academic achievement) between the genders and different ethnic groups are the consequence of some underlying biological factor or the result of environmental influences. All three of these studies come down firmly on the nurture side of this debate. Mellanby, for example, suggests that there are no real differences between the genders except for relatively minor ones in measured verbal ability, so the fact that male students get higher classification degrees from Oxford University than female students indicates some inherent bias in the awarding system. Similarly, the study on talk, gender and teachers' questioning in English lessons implies that teachers' covert biases may affect the way they assess students and, therefore, the achievement of those students.

Usefulness

A number of suggestions for the way that teachers are trained can be made from the above studies. The Mellanby *et al.* study, for example, suggests that teachers need to be trained to set up assessment systems and mechanisms that do not discriminate on the basis of gender. This training should certainly include raising the awareness of the teachers' own covert biases, as shown in the study on talk, gender and teachers' questioning in English lessons. Based on the findings of the Cline *et al.* study, teachers should also be trained and resources developed for the introduction of a multicultural dimension into the curriculum. As they point out in their study, almost every teacher in England will teach students from ethnic minorities to one degree or another and awareness of and sensitivity to cultural differences will ensure that such students are not systematically discriminated against and so will be more able to realize their potential.

EDUCATION
Learning and teaching styles

STUDY 15
Brand, S., Dunn, R., Greb, F., 2002, 'Learning styles of students with Attention Deficit Hyperactivity Disorder: who are they and how can we teach them?', *The Clearing House*, 75, 5, 268–74

Aim   To investigate whether children with ADHD have different learning styles.

Method   A quasi-experiment.

Participants   230 students (187 male, 43 female) in primary and secondary schools in New York and New Jersey. All the participants were being medically treated for ADHD, had volunteered for the study and were ensured of confidentiality.

Procedure   In both the primary and secondary school groups, age- and grade-appropriate versions of the Dunn and Dunn Learning Style Inventory (LSI) were used to identify each participant's learning style. In particular, the researchers assessed each individual's reactions to 21 elements while they were focusing on new and challenging academic knowledge or skills. The elements included reaction to the surrounding environment (silence versus noise, bright versus soft lighting, temperature differences and seating arrangements), their emotionality (motivation, persistence, preference for guidance versus choice etc.) and social preferences for learning (alone, small groups, with an adult rather than peers etc.). The LSI is known to be a valid and reliable measure of learning style.

Results   Among the primary school pupils it was found that a large number (but by no means all of them) preferred to work in low light and in the afternoon rather than in bright light and in the morning. It was also found that they generally lacked persistence and this was more characteristic of girls than boys. The data also indicated that these children were more motivated by their parents than their non-ADHD diagnosed school peers. The authors point out that these findings reject their null hypothesis that predicted that there would be no common learning style characteristics in this group.

Among the secondary school students, a preference for afternoon lessons that were highly structured with information presented in patterns was found. They also indicated a preference for a more kinaesthetic approach to learning, and this was especially true of the boys. This group was also more highly motivated by their parents than the general school population.

STUDY 16
Skogsberg, K., Clump, M., 2003, 'Do psychology and biology majors differ in their study processes and learning styles?', *College Student Journal*, 37, 1, 27–34

| Aim | To investigate whether or not psychology and biology majors have different learning styles. Previous research had shown that psychology students experienced more difficulty in studying biology than psychology and vice versa for biologists, and this study was conducted to try to see if differences in learning style could account for this. |

| Method | A quasi-experiment. |

| Participants | 87 undergraduate students (70 per cent female) who were studying psychology as their major subject and biology as a minor component of that course and 92 undergraduate students (55 per cent female) who were studying biology as their major subject and psychology as a minor component. The age range of the participants was 18–47 years (mean = 23.88 years, SD = 6.19). |

| Procedure | All the participants were required to complete the Biggs, Kember and Leung two-factor Revised Study Process Questionnaire (R-SPQ-2F). This learning styles inventory, rather than attempting to identify predetermined or permanently ingrained learning styles for groups of students, evaluates how students approach the study of the subjects most important to them. Additionally, by changing the wording in the instructions, it can be used to evaluate a student's learning style in relation to specific courses or topics. |

The R-SPQ-2F consists of 20 self-report items that categorize students as possessing a Deep Approach or a Surface Approach to studying. Each of these approaches contains two sub-scales: Motive and Strategy. The Deep Approach Scale is focused on intrinsic factors (such as developing understanding and satisfaction), while the Shallow Approach is focused on extrinsic factors (such as fear of failure and amount of effort needed to complete a task).

The inventory is completed by the participants responding to each of the 20 items via a 5-point Likert scale (1 = never or rarely true of me, 5 = always or almost always true of me).

The R-SPQ-2F was handed out to the participants to be completed either during a lecture or a lab class. They were instructed to answer each question as honestly as possible and to indicate their usual way of studying when completing the questionnaire.

| Results | There were no significant differences between the two groups in terms of the Surface Approach scale, but the psychologists showed a greater preference for the Deep Approach than did the biology students. |

STUDY 17

Curtner-Smith, M. D., Todorovich, J. R., McCaughtry, N. A., Lacon, S. A., 2000, 'Influence of the National Curriculum for Physical Education on inner-city teachers' use of teaching styles', *Research Quarterly for Exercise and Sport*, 71, 1, 68

Aim

To investigate whether or not, four years after the introduction of the English and Welsh National Curriculum for Physical Education (NCPE), teachers had developed an expanded range of teaching styles to deliver the planning, performance and evaluation of movement by pupils that the NCPE required.

Method

Experiment, with data from a previous similar study that was conducted shortly after the introduction of the NCPE (Curtner-Smith and Hasty, 1997) being used as a control group.

Participants

18 PE teachers from seven state comprehensive schools in a large city in south-east England.

Procedure

Two lessons in which a sports activity was being taught were videotaped. The teachers decided which lessons would be recorded. The lessons selected were aimed at teaching typical British summer sports such as athletics, tennis and cricket. The lessons were then analysed by the researchers using the Instrument for Identifying Teaching Styles (IFITS), a systematic observation instrument designed to record the percentage of time teachers utilize the teaching styles described by Mosston in 1981. These styles are shown in the table below:

Teaching style		Defining characteristic
Direct	1. Command	All decisions are made by the teacher
	2. Practice	Students carry out teacher-prescribed movement tasks
	3. Reciprocal	Students work in pairs on teacher-prescribed tasks: one student acts, the other provides feedback
	4. Self-check	Teacher plans and students monitor their own performance against criteria
	5. Inclusion	Planned by teacher, students monitor personal progress
Indirect	6. Guided discovery	Teacher provides assistance to solving movement problems
	7. Problem-solving	Students find answers to problems set by the teacher without assistance
	8. Individual	Teacher sets content, student plans programme
	9. Learner-initiated	Student plans programme, teacher acts as advisor
	10. Self-teaching	Student is teacher and learner, takes responsibility for own learning

Results

The 18 PE teachers spent 78 per cent of their time using direct teaching styles, with 73 per cent of their time spent utilizing the practice style. Only 5 per cent of their time was used in indirect teaching, with 4 per cent being spent using guided discovery. The teachers in the present study used the practice style to a significantly higher degree than in the previous study.

STUDY 18

Farkas, R. D., 2003, 'Effects of traditional versus learning-styles instructional methods on middle school students', *The Journal of Educational Research*, 97, 1, 42–53

Aim

To investigate whether or not teaching about the Holocaust using learning-styles instructional methods will improve student achievement, student attitudes towards teaching, student empathy towards others and student transfer task scores compared to using traditional teaching methods.

Method

An independent measures experiment.

Participants

105 seventh-grade pupils in a New York school, with a mean age of 12 years. They were in four classes, with two classes allocated to the control condition and two to the experimental condition. The participants in each of the four classes were similar in terms of educational ability, class, ethnicity and level of parental education.

Procedure

For this study, data was gathered using four instruments:
1) Dunn and Dunn's Learning Styles Inventory (LSI), to identify preferred learning style
2) a semantic differential scale that measured attitudes towards the teaching received
3) the Balanced Emotional Empathy Scale (BEES), which measured empathy towards others
4) the Moral Judgement Inventory (MJI), which measured stages of moral development and transfer of knowledge.

The LSI was administered at the outset of the study and the participants in the experimental condition were grouped according to their learning style. No such grouping occurred for the control condition. Additionally, all participants were pre-tested for their knowledge of the Holocaust and the BEES was also administered prior to teaching taking place.

The participants then undertook a teaching programme about the Holocaust, which entailed a 42-minute lesson every schoolday for 20 consecutive days. The control group were taught using traditional methods. The experimental group were taught using a Multisensory Instructional Package (MIP), which consists of a set of resources allowing the teaching of the same content in a way that maps to the learning styles identified in the LSI. Thus visual and tactual students who tend to require structure used a Programmed Learning Sequence; motivated visual and auditory learners used a Contract Activity Package; tactual students also used Task Cards, Flip Chutes and Electroboards; and kinaesthetic learners used floor games. The same teacher took all four classes.

At the end of the teaching programme, the teacher administered the BEES and MJI. The students were also given another test about the Holocaust and the semantic differential scale on attitudes to teaching to complete.

Results	

The students who received the learning-styles approach teaching showed a significantly greater increase in their knowledge of the Holocaust (as measured by the difference between their pre- and post-content test scores) than the control group. The experimental group also showed a significantly more positive attitude towards the teaching they had received than did the control group. Similarly, the change in the degree of empathy towards others, as measured by the differences in their BEES scores, was significantly greater in the experimental group than in the control group. Finally, there was also a significant difference in the MJI scores of the two groups, with the experimental group being far more able to transfer knowledge from one context to another than the control group.

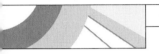

Evaluating research into learning and teaching styles

Reliability and validity

Any research into learning and teaching styles inevitably involves making some form of assessment of these two variables. For that research to have any real meaning, it is important that the measurements made of learning and teaching styles are reliable and valid. For example, if the measurements taken in the Brand et al., Skogsberg and Clump and Farkas studies are not reliable and valid, then the conclusions that can be drawn from them about how best to teach students with different learning styles will not be reliable either. The fact that these studies used inventories which have been shown, via research, to be both reliable and valid gives greater strength to the conclusions that learning styles of students should be taken into account by teachers when they draw up their schemes of work, lesson plans and resource lists.

Ecological validity

By conducting research using real teachers and students in real school/college settings, all the studies summarized above can be said to have a high degree of ecological validity. This is vitally important since, if research into psychology and education is to have any usefulness, it is important that it relates as directly as possible to the everyday experience of those who inhabit the world of education i.e. the students and teachers. Thus the Curtner-Smith et al. study into the teaching styles of PE teachers in response to the National Curriculum for PE in England and Wales gives a valid picture of what PE teaching is actually like rather than what educationalists claim it should be. Similarly, the study by Brand et al. on the learning styles of children with ADHD is important as it highlights differences in learning styles between such children, one of which – their preference for afternoon and early evening study – is at direct odds with the way the school system is currently organized.

Ethics

While we can assume that those who volunteer for research, as they did in the Brand et al., Skogsberg and Clump and Curtner-Smith et al. studies are, by that act, giving their consent to take part, there are other ethical issues that are far more important. At the outset of research, psychologists formulate hypotheses in which they predict the likely outcome(s) of their research. This prediction is based on a great deal of previous research that they read through prior to formulating their hypothesis. Thus they are reasonably confident about the way their study will turn out. This means, for instance, that Farkas was very aware that students in the learning-styles approach group would be far more likely to benefit from the study she conducted than those in the traditional teaching group. One could argue that the least the researcher could do then is to apply the experimental treatment to the control group as well, in order to compensate for them not receiving it in the first place. On the other hand, as it was only for four weeks, it may not have had any lasting effect. Moreover, in the greater scheme of things, it could be argued that if the findings of this study are applied to teaching about the Holocaust and other such sensitive and important issues in the future, then the small amount of disadvantage placed on the 50 or so participants in the control condition of Farkas's study is outweighed by the benefit to be derived by future students as a consequence.

Usefulness

Each of the above studies has important implications for how we educate students. Although only one of the studies – the Curtner-Smith *et al.* study on the teaching styles of PE teachers – involved teachers as participants, they all have points to make about the way that teachers are trained and how they teach. All four studies indicate, to some degree, that an understanding of the relationship between teaching style and learning style is important to effective learning. It could even be argued that the three studies which used students as participants effectively come to the same conclusion – teachers must make steps towards accommodating different learning styles in the way they prepare for and deliver lessons if they are to avoid systematically disadvantaging students they teach. In addition to this, the Farkas study suggests that by doing this, not only will students learn and achieve more, they will also become more empathic and rounded human beings. Thus the inclusion of learning and teaching styles in the curriculum of trainee teachers is, these studies would suggest, a cornerstone for successful education.

STUDY 19
Dolezal, S. E., Welsh, L. M., Pressley, M., Vincent, M. M., 2003, 'How nine third-grade teachers motivate student academic engagement', *The Elementary School Journal*, 103, 3, 239–69

Aim

To investigate how teachers motivate learners.

Method

Observation and interview.

Participants

Nine experienced female teachers in eight Catholic junior schools. Informed consent was obtained.

Procedure

Data were gathered via classroom observations. There were three observations, each taking one hour, of each teacher per month. The teachers were observed until no new data were found. Observers sat in unobtrusive areas of the classroom and had very little interaction with the teachers or students. Infrequently, when the children had been set work to do (i.e. they were not receiving direct instruction or assistance from the teacher), they would ask clarifying questions of the teachers or walk around the classroom to observe whether or not the children were carrying out the task they had been set by the teacher. Data were gathered in note form and each researcher drew up their own categories as the study progressed. When all the observations had been completed, the researchers came together and agreed on a common set of categories that would allow them to classify the teachers as low, moderate or high in terms of how engaging they were.

At the end of the academic year all the teachers were interviewed using a semi-structured approach to clarify questions about their teaching style and their beliefs about teaching. The teachers were encouraged to provide as much detail as they wanted. The interviews were tape-recorded and notes were taken during the interview itself. These data were then combined with those from the observations to ensure that the teachers had been appropriately classified.

Throughout the study examples of student work were collected and combined with the classroom observations of their behaviour, and this was contrasted with the degree of engagement shown by the teachers.

Results

Low-engaging teachers – students in these classes exhibited a great deal of inattention, spent a great deal of time off-task and generally did not participate in lessons. The classrooms of low-engaging teachers were sparsely decorated, with few, if any, examples of student work on display. The most prominent feature in such classrooms was a list of rules and the punishments for breaking those rules. Such teachers also had poor classroom management skills and often resorted to shouting as a means of controlling the students' behaviour. Generally, lessons were poorly planned and little positive feedback given to students and there was no use of scaffolding to allow understanding to develop. Additionally, students were generally given work that was unchallenging for them to complete. Students in such classes showed a low level of achievement and little self-regulating behaviour. They were poorly motivated to learn.

Moderately engaging teachers – these were more positive towards their students than the low-engaging teachers. They enthusiastically supported student achievement and the use of scaffolding was apparent. The classroom layout was organized to promote cooperation, exploration and student participation. The walls of the classroom showed examples of student work and a great deal of positive reinforcement was used. These teachers used a classroom management system centred on the everyday routines and procedures of the class. This meant that the students knew what they were supposed to do and when and consequently they exhibited a high level of self-regulation. At times, however, the students did go off-task and some disruptive behaviour was observed. The researchers put this down to the fact that, in the main, the level of work set for the students was not challenging enough. Thus while the students were moderately motivated to learn, there were occasions when they were not.

Highly engaging teachers – the creation of warm, caring learning environments which challenged students, supported them in risk-taking and developed their cognitive skills were the main characteristics of this group of teachers. Discriminative use of positive reinforcement, combined with complex, challenging yet ultimately achievable work was combined with very thoroughly planned lessons that minimized the opportunity for disruptive and off-task behaviour. When such behaviour did occur it was dealt with quickly and quietly, with the teacher redirecting the student back to the task in hand in a supportive manner. Each child was targeted with support that met their needs and all children were enthusiastic about learning. There was a high degree of peer support and student work was prominently displayed.

In summary, the appropriate use of positive reinforcement, stimulating, challenging yet achievable tasks, individual attention and celebration of achievement results in highly motivated students.

STUDY 20

Martinez, R., Sewell, K. W., 2000, 'Explanatory style as a predictor of college performance in students with physical disabilities', *The Journal of Rehabilitation*, 66, 1, 30–40

Aim	To investigate the role of explanatory style in the educational performance of students with physical disabilities. In particular, it was hypothesized that students with a pessimistic explanatory or attributional style would achieve less, generate more global/less specific academic goals and be less likely to rate themselves as achieving those goals than those with a more optimistic style. The study also investigated whether or not there would be differences in the above between students with/without physical disabilities.
Method	A quasi-experiment.
Participants	38 university students with physical disabilities – hearing impairment (n = 7), sight impairment (n = 10), hidden impairment (n = 5) and motor/skeletal impairment (n = 16) – and 32 university students without physical disabilities. The students were matched on age (mean = 32 years), academic ability, length of time in higher education, number of hours per week they attended courses and socio-economic status. If appropriate, students were rewarded with extra credit for their courses for participating. Informed consent was obtained from the volunteers.
Procedure	The students were given three inventories to measure relevant variables, which they completed individually at home. The Academic Goals Questionnaire was used to assess the specificity of the academic goals that students set themselves and their beliefs about whether or not they would achieve them. The students had to create a list of up to five academic goals and independent raters applied a scale from 1 (general e.g. to improve) to 4 (specific e.g. to obtain a mark of x on next assignment), depending on how specific the goals were. The mean of these was used for analysis. Likelihood of achieving them was measured on a scale from 0 (not at all) to 100 (very confident).

The Academic Attributional Style Questionnaire (AASQ) was used to measure explanatory or attributional style. This is a 36-item questionnaire in which respondents have to give a single cause for 12 negative education-related events. Each cause is then rated on a 7-point Likert scale in terms of that cause being external/internal, unstable/stable and specific/global. These scores are then averaged and the higher the score, the more pessimistic the explanatory style.

The final inventory was the revised version of the Beck Depression Inventory, which is a 21-item questionnaire measuring depression. The higher the score, the more severe the depression. This was undertaken so that a statistical control for depression could be applied to the data analysis.

The participants were given and completed the questionnaires in a medium with which they were comfortable. For example, some of those with visual impairment used large-print versions, while others used audio versions and some returned their responses on audio cassette or Braille.

Additionally, the researchers, with the participants' agreement, obtained data (Grade Point Average – GPA) on their academic performance from university authorities.

| Results |

Negative associations were found between scores on the AASQ and GPA, such that the more pessimistic the explanatory style, the lower the academic performance of the students. This held true even when depression was controlled for.

It was also found that the more pessimistic the explanatory style, the more specific the goals and the lower the rating on the likelihood of achieving those goals.

No significant differences were found between the students with physical disabilities and the students with no physical disabilities.

> **STUDY 21**
> House, J. D., 2003, 'The motivational effects of specific instructional strategies and computer use for mathematics learning in Japan: findings from the Third International Mathematics and Science Study (TIMSS)', *International Journal of Instructional Media*, 30, 1, 77–98

Aim

To investigate the effects of different teaching strategies on the motivation of Japanese mathematics students.

Method

Correlation.

Participants

10,271 Japanese maths students aged 13 years. They were selected using a two-stage cluster sampling method. First, a number of schools were randomly selected from a directory of all the schools in Japan. Second, a number of classes were randomly selected from each selected school.

Procedure

The students were asked to complete a questionnaire to assess the effects of two instructional or teaching strategies on their level of motivation for learning maths. The two teaching strategies were teaching activities used for new topic areas and typical classroom teaching activities.

The former was measured by asking the students questions about how often their teacher explained the rules and definitions, used practical or story problems related to everyday life, instructed them to work in pairs or small groups on a problem, asked what they knew about the topic at the outset, instructed them to look at the textbook while the teacher talked about it and asked them to try to solve an example related to the new topic area.

Typical teaching activities were measured by asking how frequently the following occurred:
1) teacher demonstrated how to solve maths problems
2) they worked individually from worksheets and/or textbooks
3) they worked on projects
4) they used computers
5) they did pair and/or small group work
6) they used everyday things to help solve maths problems.
For both variables frequency was measured on a 4-point scale (1 = almost always, 4 = never).

Motivation for learning maths was measured by asking the students to rate on a 4-point scale (1 = strongly agree, 4 = strongly disagree) the extent to which they agreed with the statement, 'I enjoy learning maths'.

Results

In relation to the teaching strategies used when introducing a new topic area, there were significant positive relationships between each of the six different teaching activities and student enjoyment of, and therefore motivation for, learning maths. Overall, a similar set of significant positive relationships was found for all the typical classroom strategies, although the use of computers was far less frequent for girls than for boys.

STUDY 22
Stefanou, C., Parkes, J., 2003, 'Effects of classroom assessment on student motivation in fifth-grade science', *The Journal of Educational Research*, 96, 3, 152–64

| Aim | To investigate the effects of different forms of assessment on students' motivation to learn science. More specifically, to investigate whether performance assessment is a better motivator of students than traditional methods of assessment. |

Aim

To investigate the effects of different forms of assessment on students' motivation to learn science. More specifically, to investigate whether performance assessment is a better motivator of students than traditional methods of assessment.

Method

Experiment with repeated measures design.

Participants

79 students aged 10–11 years, from three science classes in the same school in a rural area of the USA. All three classes were taught by the same teacher. 58 per cent of the sample was male, 35 per cent was female and the gender of the remaining 7 per cent was not recorded.

Procedure

All the classes followed the same science units and were assessed at the end of each one. The assessments were counterbalanced across the three classes and the three units. The three forms of assessment were:
1) a traditional paper and pencil test, involving items such as multiple choice, true/false, matching, fill in the blank and short essays
2) a traditional laboratory assessment
3) a performance assessment developed from the traditional laboratory assessment. The classroom teacher devised the paper and pencil test and the researcher, in conjunction with the teacher, devised the laboratory and performance assessments.

Students' motivation was measured via the 12-item Science Attitudes, 12-item Goal Orientations and 15-item Cognitive Engagement sub-scales of the Science Activity Questionnaire. The higher the score on the Science Attitudes sub-scale, the more favourable a student's attitude towards science is said to be. High scores on the Goal Orientations sub-scale indicate more mastery-learning goal orientations, while high scores on the Cognitive Engagement sub-scale reflect more self-regulated and engaged learning behaviours. These measures were taken after each of the three assessments.

A few days after the third assessment, the researchers held classroom discussions with each class to gather some qualitative data. In particular, they asked which type of assessment the students had preferred, how the performance assessment could be made worth taking and if their assessment preference would change if grades were not a factor.

Results

Data from 22 students were excluded from analysis as they were absent from school on the day that either the laboratory or performance assessments were held. As these were based on group tasks, it was not possible to do them at a later point.

The quantitative data indicated that goal orientation may be influenced by assessment type, since both paper and pencil and performance assessments resulted in mastery-goal orientations being reported. There was no influence of assessment type on the other two variables of attitudes to science and cognitive engagement.

The qualitative data indicated that the students were very concerned with grades and, for that reason, preferred the traditional paper and pencil tests as they were familiar with them and believed that they would help them better achieve their target grades. When asked which form of assessment they would prefer if grades were not involved, many more students opted for the performance assessment as they found it more stimulating and challenging than the paper and pencil test.

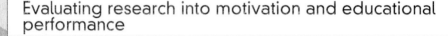

Evaluating research into motivation and educational performance

Determinism and free will

One of the major philosophical debates that runs through psychology is the determinism/free will debate. Determinists argue that all human behaviour has an explainable cause over which we exert little or no influence. Proponents of free will, however, argue that human behaviour is the result of choices and decisions that we make and that we are free to act in any number of possible ways. Thus if someone is academically motivated, determinists would seek to find a cause for that motivation. It could be argued that the four studies described above all come down on the determinist side of the debate. The Dolezal *et al.* study on engaging teachers, for example, implies that the extent to which students are motivated is determined by how engaging the teacher is and, since students can rarely choose their teacher, they have no control over how motivated they will be. Interestingly, this study does not tell us what motivates the teachers to be low-, moderately or highly engaging. Similar examples of environmental determinism (i.e. where the cause of behaviour lies in some external event or process) can be seen in the House study of maths students in Japan and the Stefanou and Parkes study on assessment and motivation. Again, it is the teaching strategies or assessment techniques used by teachers that determine whether or not their students are motivated to learn. The Martinez and Sewell study, however, while supporting the determinist point of view, suggests that motivation is the result of a cognitive process – explanatory style, and so is an example of internal determinism. This form of determinism is based on a major assumption of the cognitive approach to human behaviour – human beings are logical, rational thinking machines, and the way that we think determines how we behave. None of the studies consider the possibility that students are motivated simply because they have chosen to be.

Quantitative and qualitative data

We live in an age where scientific proof is generally accepted as revealing the true state of things. In order to prove something scientifically, you need to carry out statistical testing in order to be able to have confidence in the rejection of the null hypothesis. To conduct statistical testing you need quantitative data, hence the use of numerical scales to measure behaviour. With the exception of the Dolezal *et al.* study, all the studies outlined above use numerical scales to measure what happens in a classroom and/or to measure students' enjoyment/motivation to learn in given subjects. While this does allow for significance testing – and that is a great strength of the quantitative approach to data – it tells us nothing about the actual experience of what it is like to be a motivated student and the reasons for that motivation. It was for this very reason that Stefanou and Parkes, in their study on assessment types and motivation, also gathered qualitative data. Via this approach they were able to discover that achievement of grades influenced children's assessment preferences, for example. Similarly, the Dolezal et al. study, which only collected qualitative data, gives far more insight into what makes a low-, moderately or highly engaging teacher, and, therefore, information about how to motivate students to learn, than scores on a scale could do.

Generalization

In a very basic sense, psychology is an attempt to explain human behaviour. In an ideal situation, the way in which this would be done would be for researchers to study every single instance of a behaviour and then draw conclusions about the causes and consequences of that behaviour from their findings. Obviously, this is impossible, so what they do instead is to study a small sample of the behaviour they are researching and attempt to generalize from that sample to the wider population. While this may seem easy to do, there are inherent difficulties in this process. For example, the fact that Dolezal et al. discovered that highly engaging teachers motivated their students more than low-engaging teachers in a very small number of Catholic junior schools does not necessarily mean that such teachers will have a similar effect elsewhere. It may be, for instance, that the whole school ethos in a Catholic school is very different from that in a non-denominational school, an Islamic school, a Church of England school and so on, and it is this, rather than how engaging the teacher is, that motivates some students. The fact that the motivated students and the engaging teacher happened to be in the same class could be coincidental. Similarly, while the House study on motivation of Japanese maths students involved a very large sample, it could be that Japanese society values maths more than other societies and so it is for cultural reasons, rather than teaching strategies, that these students are motivated. Similar points can be made about our ability to generalize from the Martinez and Sewell study on explanatory styles and the Stefanou and Parkes study on the effects of different assessment types on students' enjoyment of/motivation for science.

Usefulness

One of the main aims of psychology is to develop an understanding of human behaviour so that it can be changed for the benefit of humankind. The way this can be achieved is through the development of applications based on research findings. In other words, the research is useful in that its findings and conclusions can be used to change the way we do things. For example, both the Dolezal et al. and the House studies draw conclusions that have implications for the way teachers are trained. They both highlight the use of a variety of different teaching strategies and the setting of appropriately challenging work as a means of motivating students to learn, and it should be feasible to incorporate this into teacher training programmes. Similarly, the Stefanou and Parkes study is useful in that it can provide guidance for teachers on how different forms of assessment affect the motivational level of their students. The Martinez and Sewell study on explanatory style in students with physical disabilities is useful in a number of ways. First, it tells us that a particular measuring instrument, the AASQ, is a valid and reliable instrument for measuring the attributional style of people with physical disabilities as well as those without physical disabilities. Second, and perhaps more importantly, it tells us that there are fewer cognitive differences between people with or without such disabilities than a lot of people think. The study also underpins the assumptions behind the Special Educational Needs and Disabilities Act (SENDA, 2001), which places legal requirements on education providers to make all reasonable attempts to accommodate the needs of people with disabilities.

STUDY 23

Mantzicopoulos, P. Y., 2000, 'Can the Brigance K&1 Screen detect cognitive/academic giftedness when used with preschoolers from economically disadvantaged backgrounds?', *Roeper Review*, 22, 3, 185–201

| Aim | To investigate whether or not the Brigance K&1 Screen can be used to reliably and validly assess giftedness in children from economically disadvantaged backgrounds. |

| Method | A correlation. |

| Participants | 134 children aged 52–69 months (mean = 61.6 months, SD = 3.37) from a Head Start pre-school programme in the midwest USA. 77 per cent were Caucasian, 19 per cent African-American and 4 per cent from other ethnic groups. They all spoke English as a first language and were all classified as being economically disadvantaged. The sample was equally divided with respect to gender. |

| Procedure | All the children were screened individually by the researchers with the kindergarten form of the Brigance K&1 Screen during their second semester in the Head Start programme. This inventory is a 12-sub-scale inventory that measures, among other things, knowledge of personal information, picture vocabulary, visual discrimination, rote counting from 1–10, syntax and fluency. It is a very easily administered test and requires little special training to administer and interpret it and hence is easy for teachers to use as part of their day-to-day assessments of children's abilities. It has been shown to be 77 per cent reliable in detecting children with disabilities and academic underachievement and 60 per cent reliable in identifying giftedness. When combined with teacher and parental ratings, its reliability for identifying giftedness increases to 80 per cent. |

In order to assess the concurrent validity of the Brigance K&1 Screen for this sample, the children were also assessed using the Kaufman Assessment Battery for Children (K-ABC). This inventory is a standardized measure that yields a Mental Processing Composite score that has concurrent validity with IQ, as measured by IQ tests such as the Stanford-Binet and Wechsler Intelligence Scales. This assessment was also conducted by the researchers at the same time as the Brigance K&1.

Concurrent validity testing was also conducted against the Peabody Picture Vocabulary Test – revised (PPVT-R). This is an achievement test which measures receptive vocabulary and has been shown to be a reliable and valid measure of educational aptitude. The PPVT-R was administered by kindergarten teachers some months after the above tests, following the children's move from Head Start to kindergarten. The PPVT-R is regularly used to identify gifted children in kindergarten, and administering it was part of the normal routine for the staff. The teachers were blind to the children's scores on the other two inventories.

| Results |

On the basis of achieving a score of 115 or more on the K-ABC, 13 children (with a mean score of 120) were identified as being gifted. Of these, seven were also identified as being gifted as a result of their scores on the PPVT-R.

All of those identified as being gifted scored significantly higher on the Brigance K&1 and on the teachers' ratings. This suggests that, if used with caution, the Brigance K&1 can be used as a tool for the early assessment of giftedness.

STUDY 24
Burke, M. D., Hagan-Burke, S., Sugai, G., 2003, 'The efficacy of function-based interventions for students with learning disabilities who exhibit escape-maintained problem behaviours: preliminary results from a single-case experiment', *Learning Disability Quarterly*, 26, 1, 15–26

| Aim | To investigate the effectiveness of using functional behavioural assessment as a basis for developing an intervention programme for a student with a learning disability who exhibited high rates of disruptive behaviours during reading lessons. |

Aim
To investigate the effectiveness of using functional behavioural assessment as a basis for developing an intervention programme for a student with a learning disability who exhibited high rates of disruptive behaviours during reading lessons.

Method
A single-participant experiment.

Participants
A third-year student in a junior school who had been diagnosed with a learning disability at the age of seven years. He was from a low-income household and spoke English as a second language, Spanish being his first. This student was selected because he had been identified by his teachers as exhibiting a high level of problem behaviours that ranged form mild off-task behaviours (such as fidgeting and quietly refusing to work) to more disruptive behaviours (such as singing loudly and arguing with teachers) that interfered with other students' learning. The teachers also thought that the majority of these behaviours were a form of avoidance mechanism with regard to reading tasks.

Procedure
The procedure fell into three parts.

First, a functional behavioural analysis (FBA) was conducted. This comprised a number of elements. A structured interview with the participant and his teachers took place, to elicit information about when and where the participant exhibited problem behaviours and what, if any, consequences of that behaviour served to maintain it. The interviews revealed that insubordination, failure to complete tasks, off-task behaviour and out-of-seat behaviour were the most frequent problem behaviours exhibited and that they occurred most frequently during reading instruction. One particular context that seemed to exacerbate the frequency of these behaviours was the reading circle in which students participated in oral reading exercises intermingled with comprehension tasks.

The second element of the FBA was a curriculum-based assessment (CBA) of the participant's reading abilities in relation to his classmates. This was done by the administration of an oral reading fluency (measured by the number of words correctly decoded per minute) and a reading comprehension test to the whole class on three occasions across the school year. The participant's oral reading fluency was found to be in line with his age and he was not considered to be at risk of failing to learn to read on this measure. His reading comprehension, however, was at the bottom of the lowest quartile and indicated that he was at risk of failing to learn to read.

This was followed by classroom observation of the participant's behaviour, utilizing an observation schedule developed on the basis of the findings from the first two elements of the FBA. Specifically, types of problem behaviour, the instructional context in which they were exhibited, associated antecedent behaviour, reinforcing consequences and the behaviour of a peer referent were all recorded. The observations reinforced the data from the interviews and the reading comprehension test, that the participant engaged in problem behaviour when confronted with a reading comprehension task (an average of 48 per cent of the time was spent off-task) and would persist with such behaviour until the work demands were reduced or removed. Thus he effectively avoided doing the work and the removal of the work helped to maintain his avoidance behaviours. When work was not removed, the behaviours escalated and he would become insubordinate and non-compliant.

The second part of the procedure was to conduct a functional analysis of the data identified in the FBA. On the basis of this analysis, an intervention programme, consisting of pre-teaching vocabulary concepts to the participant prior to in-class reading lessons, was developed. It was considered that such an intervention would provide the participant with sufficient prior knowledge for him to be able to complete the reading comprehension tasks effectively.

The third part of the procedure was to implement the intervention programme. To do this a repeated measures design was used. On some days the participant would receive the pre-teaching of vocabulary concepts before reading lessons in class and on other days he did not. The effect of these two conditions on the amount of time the participant spent on-task with no disruptive or other problem behaviours was measured.

| Results |

In reading comprehension tasks which were preceded by the pre-teaching of vocabulary concepts an average of 99 per cent of the time was spent on-task, compared with 38 per cent without the pre-teaching.

STUDY 25

Gillies, R. M., Ashman, A. F., 2000, 'The effects of cooperative learning on students with learning difficulties in the lower elementary school', *Journal of Special Education*, 34, 1, 19–34

| Aim | To investigate the effects of structured and unstructured group activities on the behaviours, interactions and learning outcomes of children with learning difficulties. |

Aim To investigate the effects of structured and unstructured group activities on the behaviours, interactions and learning outcomes of children with learning difficulties.

Method An experiment with independent measures design.

Participants 152 children (mean age = 9 years) from 25 classes in 11 different schools in Brisbane, Australia participated in this study, but a sub-sample of 22 of them (12 boys, ten girls) who had been diagnosed as having learning difficulties were the focus of this study.

Procedure On the basis of a cognitive ability test – the Otis-Lennon School Ability Test (OLSAT) – the 152 participants were divided into 38 gender-balanced groups of four. The allocation to these groups was done on a stratified sampling basis, such that each group had one student from the upper quartile, two from the second and third quartiles and one from the bottom quartile. The students with learning difficulties were all in the bottom quartile. Half the groups were then allocated to the structured group work condition and half to the unstructured group work condition.

Over the next six weeks, for three sessions per week (each lasting one hour), all the students followed the same social studies unit, for which their teachers had prepared group tasks and activities that required collaborative working in order to complete them.

Prior to the commencement of this, the students in the structured group condition were given two training sessions of one hour on group work skills. These sessions focused on such things as breaking tasks into components, accepting individual responsibility for completing one's own component, encouraging group involvement, sharing resources and information, listening skills, providing constructive feedback, fair task allocation and so on. The unstructured group condition did not receive this training, but were given the same two sessions of one hour to discuss how they would work as a group.

During the six-week group work activity the students were videotaped and two observers, who were blind to the study, coded their behaviour using an observation schedule. The schedule included categories for cooperative and non-cooperative behaviour, individual on-/off-task behaviour and student interactions (e.g. giving directives, giving solicited/unsolicited explanations and interruptions). Inter-observer reliability was established at 90–95 per cent for behaviour and 85–90 per cent for verbal interactions.

Learning outcomes were measured in two ways. First, the students' knowledge and understanding of the content of the social studies unit was measured via a comprehension test. They were given a score between 1 and 6 (1 = basic factual recall, 6 = complex evaluative response), depending on how they answered the questions. Second, they took an individually administered, standardized, graded word reading test, consisting of 100 words increasing in reading difficulty. The test was administered before the start of the group work sessions and again at the end so that any change in vocabulary could be measured. One point is awarded for each word correctly read.

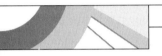

Results

There was no significant difference in the amount of cooperative behaviour shown by those children with learning difficulties in the structured and unstructured groups, but those in the latter condition exhibited significantly more off-task behaviour, suggesting that they had become less involved with their group.

It was also found that those in the structured group condition gave significantly more directions to their peers and were more helpful towards them than their counterparts in the unstructured groups.

In relation to learning outcomes, it was found that the students with learning difficulties in the structured groups scored significantly higher on the comprehension test than those in the unstructured groups, but there was no difference in their scores on the graded reading test.

Evaluating research into special educational needs

Reliability and validity

If the education system is to be in a proper position to meet the special needs of gifted students and students with learning disabilities, it is crucial that the assessment of these abilities/disabilities is valid and reliable. To achieve this, educational psychologists utilize a wide range of psychometric tests and, as part of their development, such instruments are tested for their reliability (consistency) and their validity (measuring what they purport to measure). It is important to realize, however, that a test may be valid and reliable for use with one population but not with another. It was precisely because Brigance K&1 Screen had never previously been used to identify gifted pre-schoolers from socio-economically disadvantaged backgrounds that Mantzicopoulos conducted concurrent validity testing of it by comparing it against other measures of academic ability for this particular group of students. Similarly, the reading comprehension and oral fluency tests in the Burke *et al.* study and the OLSAT comprehension and graded word reading tests in the Gillies and Ashman study had all been previously assessed for reliability and validity, and their use lends confidence to the results of the studies as being an accurate reflection of the changes they reported.

Generalization

One of the biggest factors preventing generalization of the findings from the sample in a study to the population from which that sample is drawn is sample size. This does not really present that much of a problem for the Mantzicopoulos study, with 134 participants, but it is increasingly problematic for the other two studies. Burke *et al.*'s study was only conducted on 22 students with learning difficulties, a relatively small sample. Moreover they do not report what type of learning difficulties the students have, which makes generalizing about the possible positive effects of cooperative working for students with learning difficulties even more problematical. On the face of it, generalization from the Gillies and Ashman single-participant study is even less likely, if not impossible. It could be argued, however, that while the results relate only to the participant in the study, the process of conducting a functional behavioural analysis (which by its very nature is aimed at individuals) in order to develop a tailored educational intervention can be generalized.

Perspectives

There are a number of different approaches to thinking about and conceptualizing human behaviour and each of these brings with it a set of basic assumptions about how and why we behave in the ways we do. The cognitive approach, for example, assumes that we are logical, rational information processors and that the way in which we process information governs the way we behave. This can be applied to the Burke *et al.* study. Cognitive psychologists would argue that the differences between the students with learning difficulties in the structured condition and those in the unstructured condition can be explained by the fact that the former had two hours of training on the 'rules' of cooperative working and, having taken this information on board, they changed their behaviour accordingly, while the latter, not having been given this information, failed to engage with their groups as much. In contrast, the Gillies and Ashman study belongs very much to the behaviourist approach. This approach argues that human behaviour is learned as a result of a number of different processes, but that they all essentially involve the influence of our social environment. Thus by observing the problem behaviours of their participant and the context in which they occur, and then modifying that via the intervention programme, they changed the behaviour.

Usefulness

Despite any problems associated with generalization, as mentioned above, all the studies have implications that go beyond any benefit accrued by the participants. The Mantzicopoulos study, for example, adds another tool to the repertoire for identifying giftedness, and if the educational system is to cater for gifted children appropriately it is important that they are identified as early as possible. Other research has shown that gifted children who are not being stretched by their education often engage in disruptive behaviours and are misdiagnosed with ADHD as a consequence. The early assessment of giftedness could prevent this. Similarly, both the Burke *et al.* and the Gillies and Ashman studies offer strategies to improve the educational experience of students with learning difficulties, and the inclusion of cooperative working (and group assessment?) and individually tailored educational interventions should certainly be considered when devising educational programmes for such students.

STUDY 26

Higgins, J. W., Williams, R. L., McLaughlin, T. F., 2001, 'The effects of a token economy employing instructional consequences for a third-grade student with learning disabilities: a data-based case study', *Education & Treatment of Children*, 24, 1, 99–105

Aim	

To investigate the effectiveness of using a token economy utilizing academic rewards on the behaviour of a student with learning disabilities.

Method	

A case study involving an experiment with a repeated measures design.

Participants	

A ten-year-old boy from a single-parent family, who had been diagnosed as having learning difficulties. His IQ score was within the normal range but he was below age level in reading and writing and exhibited high rates of multiple disruptive behaviours.

Procedure	

Three disruptive behaviours were targeted for intervention in this study – inappropriate talking, poor seat posture and out-of-seat behaviour, as they had been selected by his teacher and classroom assistant as the most problematical. The study was conducted in the boy's usual classroom, in which there were a further 19 students.

Baseline measures of the three disruptive behaviours were taken at the outset via observations for a number of 20-minute periods over 15 days. The frequency of occurrence of each behaviour was recorded at the end of every minute of the 20-minute period. To allow for ease of observation and to minimize disruption to the rest of the class, the boy was moved to a position on the fringe of the class. The observer was sat approximately 2 feet behind and to the right of the participant.

In the experimental condition, the participant was immediately given a tick in a box if he had not displayed any of the target disruptive behaviours in the previous minute. A grid, into which the ticks were placed, was taped to the participant's desk, thus enabling him to gain instant feedback. At the end of each session the ticks were counted up and divided by two. The figure then arrived at equated to the number of minutes available for the use of secondary reinforcements such as maths worksheets, computer time, one-to-one reading instruction, leisure reading and playing work-related games. The participant was allowed to engage in these in the first ten minutes of the following day, which was usually taken up with registration and other administrative matters, to ensure that he did not miss out on any teaching. This period of the study lasted for 12 days.

Ten to 12 days after the end of the use of the token economy, the boy was observed again to see whether or not the intervention had any lasting effects.

To ensure that the observer was recording the correct behaviours, inter-rater reliability testing was conducted, with the participant's teacher also recording the disruptive behaviours twice each during the baseline assessment and four times each during the token economy phase. Reliability was established to be 100 per cent.

| Results |

The results of the study are shown in the table below:

Observation period	Disruptive behaviours (mean frequency of occurrence)		
	Inappropriate talking	Out-of-seat behaviour	Poor seat posture
Baseline	6.0	1.9	11.0
Token economy	0.8	0.2	5.0
Maintenance	0	0	2.5

The results show that the use of a token economy reduced the occurrence of disruptive behaviours and, moreover, that this reduction was maintained after the withdrawal of the token economy.

STUDY 27

Self-Brown, S. R., Mathews, S., II, 2003, 'Effects of classroom structure on student achievement goal orientation', *The Journal of Educational Research*, 97, 2, 106–13

| Aim | To investigate the effects of different classroom assessment structures on student achievement goal orientation. It was hypothesized that the use of a token economy would lead to the setting of performance goals, the use of contingency contracting would lead to the setting of learning goals and not using either of these strategies would not differentiate the type of goals being set. |

Method   An experiment.

Participants   71 students from three different classes in a single primary school. The classes were randomly allocated to the three conditions. A fifth-year class of 25 students was allocated to the token economy condition, a fourth-year class of 18 students was allocated to the contingency contract condition and a class of 28 fifth-year students formed the control condition.

Procedure   Students in the token economy group were given a contract which explained how and at what rate tokens could be earned (e.g. four play dollars for each A or B in maths) and the secondary reinforcers (sweets, computer time, pens, keyrings) that the tokens could be exchanged for. This contract was in a folder that was kept on the students' desks. Also in the folder was a goals chart. This chart contained a list of student behaviours that could earn tokens and the number of tokens each behaviour would be rewarded with, as well as a column in which the students could record their weekly and long-term goals for maths.

Those in the contingency contract condition received a contingency contract which described how they would meet weekly with the researcher to set and discuss goals for maths. They, too, were given a folder with the contract in it to keep on their desks. The folder also contained a goals chart on which they could write their weekly and long-term maths goals. A gold star was placed next to a goal when it had been achieved.

Students in the control condition received only a goals chart on which to record their weekly and long-term maths goals.

For all students the setting of goals was done in a weekly meeting with the researcher. For the token economy and contingency contracting condition this involved discussion about these goals. In addition, it was during this meeting that the students in the token economy condition could exchange their tokens for the secondary reinforcers. For students in the control condition, no discussion, feedback or any information about their goals was provided; they simply used the time with the researcher to write their goals on their own.

The experiment was conducted over a five-week period and was in place for all maths lessons (which were conducted as they had been prior to the start of the experiment) during that time.

The students' goals were classified as either performance or learning goals by the researcher on the basis of a goal typology developed by Dweck.

Results

The results of the study are shown in the table below:

Goal type	Condition (mean goals set)		
	Token economy	Contingency contract	Control
Learning goals	0.75	14.27	5.36
Performance goals	4.95	5.55	5.61

The results uphold the experimental hypotheses that a token economy would lead to the setting of more performance than learning goals, contingency contracting would lead to the setting of more learning than performance goals and providing neither of these would not differentiate between the types of goals set.

STUDY 28
Aleven, V., Koedinger, K. R., 2002, 'An effective metacognitive strategy: learning by doing and explaining with a computer-based Cognitive Tutor', *Cognitive Science*, 26, 2, 147–79

| Aim | To investigate whether self-explanation can be scaffolded effectively in a classroom through the use of a Cognitive Tutor, a piece of intelligent instructional software that supports guided learning by doing and explanation. While this paper reports two experiments, only one will be summarized here. |

Aim To investigate whether self-explanation can be scaffolded effectively in a classroom through the use of a Cognitive Tutor, a piece of intelligent instructional software that supports guided learning by doing and explanation. While this paper reports two experiments, only one will be summarized here.

Method Experiment with a matched pairs design.

Participants 41 students of 15–16 years, from a suburban high school near Pittsburgh, PA, USA, who were studying a geometry unit on angles via one hour of teaching per week, with a second hour spent solving problems using geometry Cognitive Tutor software on a computer. Data on only 24 participants are used for analysis as some failed to complete the course in the allotted time and the teacher forgot to administer a post-experimental test to measure outcomes for others.

Procedure Before the experiment commenced the students were matched on their prior achievement on this course and this was used to allocate them to conditions. Before the start of the angles unit they were given a pre-test to assess their knowledge and understanding of angles. This acted as the baseline measurement for the effects of the two conditions.

The students were then required to work through the same geometrical problems on a computer over the course of the unit, which ran for a semester.

The two conditions in this experiment were the explanation condition and the problem-solving condition. The students in the explanation condition used a version of the Cognitive Tutor that required them to input an explanation for each step in their problem-solving process. Feedback is then given on both their solutions to the problems and their explanations. The students in the problem-solving condition (effectively the control condition) used a version of the software that did not require this input of explanations. The unit was deemed to be finished when the students met the Cognitive Tutor's predetermined criterion for mastery.

At the end of the unit a post-test to measure their knowledge and understanding of the unit content was given to the students. The differences between the scores on the pre- and post-tests were used as a measure of how much learning had been acquired by the students in each condition.

Results First, it was found that the explanation condition spent more, but not significantly more, time working on the computer than the problem-solving condition, but this was to be expected as they had an additional task (inputting their explanations) to do.

In terms of the differences between their pre- and post-test scores, the students in the explanation condition exhibited a significantly greater improvement than those in the problem-solving condition. The former also needed fewer problems to reach the Cognitive Tutor's mastery criterion than did the latter (102 versus 136 respectively).

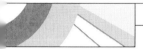

Evaluating research into perspectives on learning

Basic assumptions about human nature

Each different perspective or approach to studying human behaviour makes certain assumptions about the causes of that behaviour. The behaviourist approach, for example, assumes that all behaviour is learned and in order to explain any behaviour we simply need to discover the learning process involved. One form of learning is operant conditioning, the basic premise of which is that we will learn to behave in certain ways if that behaviour brings about pleasant consequences for us. At the same time, we will cease to behave in certain ways if that behaviour brings about negative consequences for us. It is these principles of operant conditioning that underlie the use of token economies and contingency contracting in the studies by Higgins *et al.* and Self-Brown and Mathews II. Both these studies support the idea that, if there are pleasant consequences to behaviour (i.e. receiving reinforcers, such as tokens or gold stars), that behaviour will be learned. Interestingly, the second of these studies suggests that different types of procedures for gaining those rewards can have different effects on schoolchildren, since the contingency contract children set themselves more learning goals than performance ones, while the opposite was true of the children in the token economy condition. It is also worth noting that the contingency contract group overall set more goals than those in the token economy, suggesting that contingency contracting is a more effective method of supporting students in setting goals than the use of a token economy.

One of the biggest criticisms of the behaviourist approach is that it gives scant regard to the cognitive abilities and skills that we have and, while they accept the idea that we can learn via operant conditioning, cognitive psychologists would argue that it is the way we process information that is the greatest influence on our behaviour. Thus in the Aleven and Koedinger study, it is not the fact that the students in the explanation condition receive feedback on their explanations which improves their performance (which would support the behaviourist approach), but the fact that the feedback helps them to clarify their thinking about the problems they are tackling (as indeed does inputting the explanations in the first place), so they are able to work through the problems more effectively than the students who are not required to explain each step of their problem solving.

Reductionism

Reductionism is the process by which a complex phenomenon, such as human behaviour, is broken down into a series of small components and, through the explanation of what happens at the component level, the complex whole is also explained. For the behaviourist approach, for example, the basic unit of behaviour is stimulus–response. The change in behaviour shown by the participant in the Higgins *et al.* study, as far as behaviourists are concerned, is explained entirely by the relationship between stimulus and response. In order to achieve more tokens, the boy stopped exhibiting disruptive behaviours. Similarly, the students in the Self-Brown and Mathews II study developed their goals in order to receive their reinforcers. In drawing these conclusions, and thereby taking a reductionist

STUDY GUIDE for OCR Psychology: A2 Level

approach, the authors of these studies are ignoring other possible causes. For example, it may be that the participant in the first study, unknown to the researchers, had been prescribed medication to control the disruptive behaviours and it was this that brought about the change they observed. Similarly, the latter study does not take into account the possibility that the type of goal set by the students may have been influenced by parental involvement rather than the experimental condition the children were allocated to.

Ecological validity

The more true to everyday life the procedures of psychological research are, the more confidence we can have in their explanations of how we behave. This is obviously important in relation to education, since the way in which teachers teach (and are trained) can and is influenced by such research. The fact that all these studies took place in real schools increases their ecological validity compared to laboratory studies, but, having said that, there are differences between them in terms of their level of ecological validity. For example, in the Self-Brown and Mathews II study, the weekly meeting with the researcher was not, strictly speaking, a part of everyday school life – it only happened for the duration of the study. Therefore, this study does not tell us about the implications of token economies versus contingency contracting as applied by teachers as part of their usual practice. The same could be said of the Higgins *et al.* study. The Aleven and Koedinger study, on the other hand, overcomes this problem, as the use of the computers was an integral part of the way in which students were taught on that course.

Usefulness

The Higgins *et al.* study has an obvious direct application to the teaching of children with learning difficulties who exhibit disruptive behaviour. This is that teachers should be trained and given the resources to identify the disruptive behaviour, institute a token economy to increase the amount of non-disruptive behaviour and thereby reduce the disruptive behaviour. Similarly, the Self-Brown and Mathews II study has implications for the way children are taught. One of these is that someone – perhaps the teacher, a student-learning manager or a classroom assistant – needs to be given time to sit down individually with each student every week to discuss their curriculum-related goals in order to better motivate the students. The Aleven and Koedinger study is useful in two areas. The first is very obvious: the use of appropriate Cognitive Tutors can improve student learning, so investment needs to be made in computers and software to ensure that all students have access to them as needed. Second, even without that access, teachers should ask students to explain how they arrive at the answers they give to problems they have been set as it is this process which the study suggests improves performance and achievement.

See also...	

Studies 67, 116, 117 and 128.

Section 2
HEALTH

STUDY 29

Sethi, A. K., Celentano, D. D., Gange, S. J., Moore, R. D., Gallant, J. E., 2003, 'Association between adherence to antiretroviral therapy and human immunodeficiency virus drug resistance', *Clinical Infectious Diseases*, 37, 8, 1112–18

Aim	

To investigate the relationship between cumulative adherence to prescribed drugs and the development of resistance to those drugs.

Method	

Correlation and longitudinal, as data were gathered a number of times over one year.

Participants	

195 people, aged 32–48 years, with HIV, who were out-patients at the Moore HIV Clinic, part of Johns Hopkins Hospital, Baltimore, MD, USA. This was a restricted cluster sample, in that participants had to meet the following criteria to be accepted into the study:

1) currently prescribed Highly Active Anti-Retroviral Therapy (HAART)
2) an HIV load of less than 500 copies/mL (a measure of viral infection)
3) no documentation of major mutations associated with HAART
4) no previous virologic failure, defined as two consecutive virus loads of greater than or equal to 500 copies/mL while receiving HAART.

Participants were paid $15 every time they visited the research centre to contribute data. Informed consent was obtained.

Procedure	

The study was carried out at the General Clinical Research Centre, next to the Moore Clinic. Participants were required to visit the research centre following any appointments they had at the clinic. A total of 1188 visits were made by the 195 participants during the year of the study (2000–1).

Cumulative adherence was measured using the formula P-M/P (where P = number of doses of HAART prescribed for the three days prior to the visit and M = number of doses missed during the three days prior to the visit) and was collected by self-report. Cumulative adherence was classified as 100 per cent, 90–99 per cent, 80–89 per cent, 70–79 per cent, 60–69 per cent and <60 per cent of doses taken. The following observations were made of visits for each of these categories respectively: 717 (60 per cent), 256 (22 per cent), 103 (9 per cent), 63 (5 per cent), 26 (2 per cent), 23 (2 per cent).

Resistance to the HAART drugs was measured by testing participants' blood HIV loads using a standardized, valid measure and was conducted by an independent, experienced tester who was blind to the aims of the study. An HIV load equal to or greater than 500 copies/mL was taken as indicating resistance to the drugs.

Data from participants was discounted if their clinician discontinued prescribing

HAART drugs, they stopped HAART of their own accord, did not attend the research centre for a period of six consecutive months or more, or died.

| Results |

Of the 195 participants, 28 (14 per cent) developed clinically significant resistance during the study, 129 (66 per cent) had complete follow-up and never developed clinically significant resistance and data from 38 (19 per cent) were discarded as a result of discontinuation of HAART by the clinician (14 patients), discontinuation of HAART by the patient (nine patients), loss to follow-up (five patients), death (six patients), transfer of care to other sites (three patients) and being sent to prison (one patient).

Cumulative adherence of 70–89 per cent showed a significant positive correlation with resistance to the HAART drugs. Cumulative adherence outside this range (whether higher or lower) did not significantly correlate with resistance. This supports previous research by Friedland and Williams (1999) that there is a bell-shaped relationship between adherence and drug resistance.

> ## STUDY 30
> Yung, C. Y., Tse, S. L. S., Chan, K. S. Y., Chow, C. K. C., Yau, C. W. S., Chan, T. Y. K., Critchley, J. A. J. H., 1998, 'Age-related decline in the knowledge of diabetes mellitus and hypoglycaemic symptoms in non-insulin-dependent diabetic patients in Hong Kong', *Age and Ageing*, 27, 3, 327–32

Aim

To investigate the relationship between age and knowledge of diabetes mellitus and hypoglycaemic symptoms and adherence to medical advice in patients with non-insulin-dependent diabetes mellitus.

Method

Natural experiment.

Participants

56 men and 70 women, aged 50–82 years (mean age = 64.3 years), with non-insulin-dependent diabetes mellitus, who were out-patients at a general district hospital diabetes clinic in Hong Kong. This was a cluster sample.

Procedure

Over a seven-week period between January and March 1995, all patients with non-insulin-dependent diabetes mellitus who gave informed consent were interviewed by one of three pharmacy students under the supervision of the two doctors in charge of the clinic. Data gathered, either from the participants or from their medical records, included age, sex, duration of and treatment for non-insulin-dependent diabetes mellitus, attendance at diabetes education classes, presence and extent of diabetic complications, previous hypoglycaemic attacks, other medical conditions, blood glucose and renal and liver function tests.

Each participant was then given two previously validated questionnaires to complete. The first was designed to measure their knowledge of their condition and adherence to medical advice. The questions were:
1) What is wrong with the blood glucose level in your blood?
2) What do the tablets or insulin do to your blood glucose?
3) Do you take your meals regularly every day?
4) What would happen if you miss a meal?
5) What would happen if you took too many tablets/injected too much insulin?
6) If you feel dizzy, hungry and sweaty, what is happening?
7) Do you carry your diabetic outpatient clinic card with you all the time?
8) What should you do if you have an attack of hypoglycaemia?
9) Do you carry sugar cubes (or sweets) with you?
10) Do your relatives know you have diabetes? (Yung *et al.* 1988)
Items 1, 2, 4, 5, 6 and 8 measure knowledge of diabetes mellitus and items 3, 7, 9 and 10 measure adherence to medical advice.

The second was designed to measure their knowledge of hypoglycaemic symptoms.

Which of the following are symptoms of hypoglycaemia? (answer yes, no or don't know)
1) sweating
2) weakness

3) palpitations
4) hunger
5) anxiety
6) speech disturbance
7) tingling lips
8) confusion
9) inability to concentrate
10) visual disturbance
11) faintness
12) sleepiness
13) headaches (Yung *et al.* 1988)

The questionnaires were read to those unable to read due to illiteracy or visual impairment and care was taken not to ask leading questions. The greater the number of 'correct' answers, the greater the participants' knowledge and adherence was taken to be.

Results

The data were non-parametric and statistical significance was measured using the Wilcoxon signed ranks test or chi squared test as appropriate at the $p < 0.05$ level.

There was a significant decline in the number of correct answers given to the questionnaire items on knowledge of diabetes as the age of the participants increased, but this same pattern was only true for items 7 and 9 on adherence to medical advice. There was also a significant decline in knowledge of the symptoms of hypoglycaemia among older patients for all items except item 7.

It was also found that previous experience of having suffered an actual hypoglycaemic attack (39 of the participants) had no effect on knowledge of the symptoms.

Patients who had never attended any diabetes education classes (23 participants) scored lower than other participants on all three dependent variables. Of those that had attended classes, the more recent their attendance had been, the higher they scored on the two questionnaires.

STUDY 31

Watt, P. M., Clements, B., Devadason, S. G., Chaney, G. M., 2003, 'Funhaler spacer: improving adherence without compromising delivery', *Archives of Disease in Childhood*, 88, 7, 579–82

| Aim | To investigate whether or not adherence to using an asthma medication inhaler can be improved by making the activity a 'fun' activity that children would want to undertake. |

Aim To investigate whether or not adherence to using an asthma medication inhaler can be improved by making the activity a 'fun' activity that children would want to undertake.

Method Experiment.

Participants A cluster sample of ten boys and 22 girls, aged 1.5–6 years (mean age = 3.2 years), who had suffered from asthma for an average of 2.2 years. All the participants were prescribed drugs (salbutamol and beclomethasone dipropionate) that were administered via an inhaler. The recommended dose of the inhalers used in this study is to take four or more 'shots' or cycles at a time. Informed consent was obtained from the parents of the children.

Procedure The study took place in Australia over a two-week period. In the first week the children used a standard inhaler (the Breath-A-Tech) to deliver their medication; during the second week they used a new inhaler (the Funhaler), which had attached 'toys' (a spinner and whistle), designed to distract the child from the drug delivery event itself and also to act as a form of self-reinforcement for using the inhaler correctly (if used correctly, the spinner span and the whistle sounded; if used incorrectly, they did not). The Funhaler was designed in such a way as to ensure that the toys did not interfere with the actual delivery of the drugs in any way and the modular design allowed for replacement of the toys with others should boredom set in.

Adherence was measured via the parents of the children completing a pre- and post-experimental questionnaire on the frequency and regularity of inhaler use.

Results Only 27 out of the 32 sets of parents completed both questionnaires and so only the data on 27 children were analysed.

The questionnaires revealed that 38 per cent of the parents administered the Funhaler more regularly than the standard inhaler and 60 per cent more children took the recommended four or more cycles per aerosol delivery when using the Funhaler compared with the standard inhaler.

STUDY 32
Sharma, S., Murphy, S. P., Wilkens, L. R., Shen, L., Hankin, J. H., Henderson, B., Kolonel, L. N., 2003, 'Adherence to the Food Guide Pyramid recommendations among Japanese Americans, Native Hawaiians, and whites: results from the multiethnic cohort study', *Journal of the American Dietetic Association*, 103, 9, 1195–9

Aim

To investigate ethnic differences in adherence to the American Food Guide Pyramid recommendations.

Method

A natural experiment.

Participants

Over 115,000 people, aged 45–75 years, from three different ethnic groups: white Americans (21,933 men, 25,303 women), Japanese Americans (25,893 men, 28,355 women) and Native Hawaiians (5979 men, 7650 women). This was a quota sample and informed consent was obtained.

Procedure

A questionnaire (the Food Frequency Questionnaire – FFQ) was designed specifically for this study. It was standardized on a sample of 60 men and 60 women, aged 45–75 years, from each of the three ethnic groups prior to use in the study. The questionnaire, which was conducted as a self-administered postal survey and sent to over 215,000 individuals between 1993 and 1996 (with 115,113 being returned), asked how often the respondents had eaten particular foodstuffs over the preceding three days. The foodstuffs on the list covered more than 85 per cent of the intake of fat, dietary fibre, vitamin A, carotenoids and vitamin C, as recommended by the Food Guide Pyramid, and were measured in servings, which were then converted to daily calorie intake (measured in kilocalories, or kcal). Traditional foods of each ethnic group were also included, irrespective of their contribution to nutrient intake.

Results

First, data from each individual ethnic group were compared with the daily recommended intake for each of the foodstuffs contained in the American Food Guide. It was found that there was little variation between the ethnic groups and their adherence to the recommendations of the American Food Guide. No one ethnic group adhered to the recommendations more than any other. It was found, however, that of those with a daily calorie intake below 1600kcal per day, irrespective of ethnicity, over 58 per cent failed to adhere to the daily number of servings, with dairy foodstuffs being the most likely to be missed out. It was also found that those with the highest daily calorie intake (more than 2800kcal per day), again irrespective of ethnicity, consumed more than three times as much alcohol, discretionary fat and added sugar than those with a calorie intake of less than 1600kcal per day.

There were some differences between the ethnic groups, however. The Native Hawaiian group had the highest daily calorie intake of the three groups and the highest mean body mass index (BMI). Japanese Americans had the lowest BMI. The Native Hawaiian group also ate more daily servings of all the food groups than the other two ethnic groups, with the exception of dairy products. Japanese American men ate two more servings per day of the grain food group than white men.

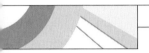

Evaluating research into adherence to medical advice

Ethics

As with all areas of health psychology, ethical considerations play a very large part in the design of a research study. Since the study is dealing with sensitive health issues, it is important that confidentiality is maintained, informed consent sought, the right to withdraw upheld, actual or potential harm minimized and so on. In this respect, all the studies outlined above can be considered ethically sound. In the Sharma *et al.* study on diet and the Watt *et al.* Funhaler study, the fact that not every participant who received the questionnaires returned them is evidence that some exercised their right to withdraw. All the studies obtained informed consent, although in the Watt *et al.* study this was gained from the parents rather than the children, due to their young age. This is acceptable within the BPS Code of Ethics, although the age at which informed consent should be obtained from the child rather than the parent is debatable. With regard to minimizing harm, the most striking example of where this was considered was the Watt *et al.* study. Prior to the study, the design of the Funhaler was carefully tested to ensure that the addition of the toys did not interfere in any way with the delivery of the asthma medication. As for the Sethi *et al.* study on HIV and the Yung *et al.* study on diabetes, it could be argued that, since they identified factors which increase non-adherence and no direct intervention was made into any medical treatment that the patients were undergoing, the implications of the studies are of positive benefit for such patients.

Reliability and validity

Whenever we attempt to measure behaviour, whether or not we are actually measuring what we think we are (validity) and whether or not we can measure it consistently (reliability) are important things to consider. Each of the above studies involves an attempt at measuring adherence to medical advice. The Sethi *et al.* study on HIV takes the most straightforward approach. Patients are asked how many doses of medication they had missed over the previous three days and their response is taken as a measure of the extent to which they adhered to medical advice. This approach has face validity: it apparently measures what it claims to measure. In fact, the use of self-reports in all the studies to ascertain the extent to which the participants took their medication or knew how to take it correctly indicates that they all possess face validity. A problem with the use of self-reports, however, is that they can lack predictive validity. Simply because a patient states that they missed x number of doses of medication over the past three days, for example, provides no basis for assuming that they will miss a similar number of doses in the future. In lacking predictive validity, the self-report approach to measuring adherence can also be said to have a low level of reliability. How accurate is the patient's recall? Can we assume that it is 100 per cent accurate? In some ways, the Yung *et al.* study on age-related factors affecting adherence to diabetic treatment regimens focuses on this very issue. The conclusion they draw about our ability to recall information related to our medical conditions and associated treatment declining as we get older suggests that we should be wary about the inferences we draw from studies in which recall is the measure of adherence.

Sampling

In an ideal world, psychological research would be conducted on all the members of a given population, since this is the only real way of being able to apply the findings of that research to that population. Unfortunately, this is not practicable; the time and expense involved in conducting research on millions of people is prohibitive. A way round this is to conduct research on a smaller subset of that population, the sample. The more characteristics the sample shares with the population, the more representative it is and the greater confidence we can have in generalizing our findings from the sample to the population. In the Sharma *et al.* study on diet and ethnicity, for example, the number of participants and their ethnicity means that we can be reasonably confident that for the ethnic groups involved there are differences in diet, but not in their adherence to the Food Guide Pyramid. We are far less able to generalize in the other three studies, however. Can we assume that the relationship between adherence to medical advice and the build-up of resistance to the prescribed drugs shown in the Sethi *et al.* study on HIV applies to other medical conditions and/or treatment regimens? After all, different drugs have different effects on the body and, perhaps more importantly, can have different effects on different people, thus limiting our ability to generalize. Despite this, it is important for researchers into medical adherence to attempt to generalize, since this can provide some indication of the factors that affect adherence rates, such as age (Yung *et al.*) and the actual experience of taking medication (Watt *et al.*), and thereby prompt suggestions for improving them and thus reducing, if not avoiding, the consequences, such as resistance to therapy (Sethi *et al.*) or the increased risk of heart disease (as implied in the Sharma *et al.* study).

Usefulness

Obviously the most useful thing about studies into adherence to medical advice is that they can reveal the reasons why people do not adhere. If this is known, health professionals are in a better position to develop strategies to improve adherence and so assist people in improving their health, recovering their health quicker or coping with chronic illness more effectively. Thus the Sharma *et al.* study provides information about adherence to diet that can be utilized by dieticians and other health professionals to develop programmes for assisting obese people in their weight-loss efforts. Additionally, research into adherence highlights the point that different groups of patients may require different approaches. This is shown by the use of the Funhaler in the Watt *et al.* study, to make taking medication an enjoyable experience for young children, and the implication of the Yung *et al.* study of the need to develop more cognitive-based strategies, such as memory aids for older people.

STUDY 33

Lysens, R. J., Ostyn, M. S., Vanden Auweele, Y., Lefevre, J., Vuylsteke, M., Renson, L., 1989, 'The accident-prone and overuse-prone profiles of the young athlete', *The American Journal of Sports Medicine*, 17, 5, 612–20

Aim	To develop a prospective accident-prone and overuse-prone profile of young athletes, i.e. to develop a tool which could be used to predict which young athletes would be more likely to suffer injury through accidents or overuse.
Method	Correlation and longitudinal, as the data was gathered over one year.
Participants	A group of 185 first-year physical education students (118 males, 67 females), aged 17–19 years, from the Catholic University of Leuven, Netherlands. This cluster sample of participants was chosen because they all follow the same sports exercise programme for 30 weeks (75 hours of gymnastics, 60 hours of track and field athletics and swimming, 37.5 hours each of basketball, handball, football and volleyball and 15 hours of dance), the playing surfaces and safety equipment are common to all and there is a standardized means of recording injuries that occur as a result of their course. Informed consent was obtained.
Procedure	All participants had to undergo a thorough medical and all existing injuries were recorded and had to be fully recovered from prior to admittance to the PE course.

To develop the profiles, a range of both physical and psychological variables was measured at the outset of the study. Anthropomorphic data included height, weight, body type (using the Heath-Carter method, a reliable and valid measure of somatotypes) and percentage of body fat (using the valid and reliable Durmin-Rahman method). Other physical characteristics, such as flexibility, limb speed, explosive strength, speed and endurance were evaluated, using the Leuven Physical Fitness Test Battery. Misalignments of feet and/or legs were also measured.

Psychological variables in the form of 16 personality traits (including neuroticism, psychosomatic stability, extroversion–introversion, self-defensiveness, social desirability, hypochondria and anxiety) were measured using six personality tests: the Spielberger State Trait Anxiety Inventory, the Bell Adjustment Inventory, the Amsterdamse Biografische Vragenlijst (based on Eysenck's two-factor theory), the Gordon Personal Profile and the Gordon Personal Inventory (which are valid Belgian equivalents of the Catell Sixteen Personality Factor Questionnaire), the California Psychological Inventory and the Eysenck Personality Inventory (EPI), often used in accident-prone studies.

A clear definition and classification of injuries sustained by the participants and a valid way of recording them was developed. An injury was defined as any injury that occurred during the sports exercise sessions and led to a minimum three-day absence from sports. The same sports doctor from the university examined and registered all injuries and made the decision as to whether the student was to cease sports activity and for how long. The types of injuries were classified into two categories: acute injuries (including contusions, sprains, dislocations and fractures) and injuries arising from overuse (including shin splints, stress fractures, tendonitis, back pain and strains). A re-injury was defined as an identical injury sustained at least one month after a participant's return to sports activities.

Results

The data revealed that 185 participants sustained 315 sports injuries (137 acute, 178 overuse) during their freshman year. The overall injury rate was 170 per 100 participant years; the frequency ratio was 4.72 injuries per student per 1000 hours of sports exercise. Injuries caused the participants to be absent from their studies for considerable periods (an average of 11 days per injury for males and 19 days per injury for females). It was found that a degree of latent hypochondria was implicated in the extent of absence. It was also found that a previous history of injury was a reliable predictor of likelihood of injuries such as sprains and stress-fractures reoccurring.

The relationships between the variables were analysed using the following contingency table and data for male and female participants were treated separately:

Injury category	Males		Females	
	Physical traits	Psychological traits	Physical traits	Psychological traits
Acute injuries (accident-prone)	Short; great upper body strength; great functional strength; high limb speed; high muscle flexibility.	Lack of caution; emotional lability; either high or low scores on the psychosomatic dimension; either high or low scores on the state anxiety dimension.	Great upper body strength; great functional strength; high body weight.	Good personal relationships; dominant; emotionally stable; lack of caution; low trait anxiety.
Overuse injuries	Tall; endomorphic; little static strength; great explosive strength; low muscle flexibility; greater Q-angle of the knee (a leg misalignment).	Sociable; extrovert; not vivacious; hypochondriacal; neurotic.	Tall; endomorphic; little static strength; great explosive strength; low muscle flexibility; greater Q-angle of the knee, leg-length discrepancy and pronated feet (leg and foot misalignments).	Vigorous; great sense of responsibility; low psychosomatic stability; neurotic.

STUDY 34
Raiche, M., Hebert, R., Prince, F., Corriveau, H., 2000, 'Screening older adults at risk of falling with the Tinetti balance scale', *The Lancet*, 356, 9234, 1001–2

Aim

To test the validity of the Tinetti balance scale as a means of predicting the likelihood of falling in older people. The Tinetti balance scale has shown good performance on inter-rater reliability and concurrent validity, but the precise score on the scale which allows health practitioners to distinguish between those at risk of falling and those not at risk has never been determined. In order to determine this score, the authors assessed the predictive validity of the Tinetti balance scale to prospectively identify those at risk.

Method

Longitudinal correlation between score on the Tinetti balance scale and number of falls over a period of one year.

Participants

225 people over the age of 75 years (mean age = 80.0 years, SD = 4.4), living in their own homes, randomly selected from the electoral roll of the urban area of Sherbrooke, Canada. Informed consent was obtained.

Procedure

The Tinetti balance scale is an observation-based way of measuring characteristics associated with falls. It assesses balance with 14 items (scored out of 24) and gait with ten items (scored out of 16) for a total score out of 40, where the lower the score, the worse the balance or gait. At the outset of the study a trained research nurse administered the Tinetti balance scale to the 225 participants in their own homes. The participants were required to carry out a series of tasks (rising from a chair, standing with eyes closed, beginning to walk and so on) and the nurses recorded a score (0, 1 or 2) for them on each of the scale items.

The participants were then given a calendar on which to record the dates of any falls they had during the coming year. Every participant was telephoned monthly and asked for the number of falls for that month. At the end of the study the number of falls was correlated with each item on the Tinetti balance scale.

Results

The mean score on the Tinetti balance scale was 33.8 (SD = 7.2). During the year 23.6 per cent (53) of the participants fell at least once and all of them scored below 33 on the scale. 120 of the 225 participants scored 36 or less. Statistical analysis showed that those scoring 36 or less had a greater than 30 per cent risk of falling, while those scoring above 36 had only a 15 per cent risk of falling. Therefore, the score of 36 was accepted as the cut-off point for predictive validity of falling. This score predicts a similar level of risk as does the Pap smear for cervical cancer, so the authors argue that this is an acceptable figure to use as a means of predicting likelihood of falling in older people and conclude that the Tinetti balance scale has predictive validity for falling.

STUDY 35

Sherry, P., Gaa, A., Thurlow-Harrison, S., Graber, K., Clemmons, J., Bobulinski, M., 2003, 'Traffic accidents, job stress and supervisor support in the trucking industry', http://www.du.edu/~psherry/trucks1.html (accessed 14 May 2004)

Aim

To study the relationship between stress and accidents in an occupational setting.

Method

A correlation in which the relationship between stress, the drivers' perceptions of their supervisors' abilities in goal setting, giving appropriate feedback and being supportive, personal attributes (distractibility, locus of control, agreeableness and risk-taking) and accidents was measured.

Participants

55 long-distance lorry drivers from a haulage company in Denver, CO, USA. Consent was obtained.

Procedure

With the exception of accidents, all of the above variables were measured by asking the participants to rate relevant items on a 5-point Likert scale (1 = to a little or no degree, 5 = to a very great degree).

The accidents variable was measured by asking three questions:
1) How many injuries have you had in the last four years?
2) How many collisions have you been involved in during the last four years?
3) How many traffic tickets have you received in the last four years?
All the items were embedded in a larger questionnaire.

Results

Initial analysis revealed a number of significant relationships between stress and injuries, between the personal attributes (distractibility, locus of control, agreeableness and risk-taking) and injuries reported and also between the drivers' perceptions of their supervisors' abilities in goal setting, giving appropriate feedback and being supportive and the number of traffic tickets received. No relationship was found between stress and number of collisions or between the personal attributes and number of collisions.

Further analysis of the relationships between the personal variables and injuries revealed that those with a low level of injury (one or no injuries in the previous four years) scored lower on the distractibility scale than those with a higher level of injury (two or more injuries in the previous four years).

STUDY 36
Gofin, R., Donchin, M., Schulrof, B., 2004, 'Motor ability: protective or risk for school injuries?' *Accident Analysis and Prevention*, 36, 43–8

| Aim | To investigate whether or not increased motor ability affected the number of accidental injuries experienced by schoolchildren. |

Aim

To investigate whether or not increased motor ability affected the number of accidental injuries experienced by schoolchildren.

Method

A natural experiment, in which it was hypothesized that children with superior motor ability would suffer fewer accidental injuries than those with lower motor ability.

Participants

2057 schoolchildren in grades 3–6 (aged 8–12 years), attending the eight different schools in a city in the north of Israel in 1995–6. Permission to conduct the study was gained from the ethics committee of the Hadassah University Hospital, the head teachers of the schools and the children's parents, who gave informed consent.

Procedure

Data on gender and grade (as a proxy for age) were gathered from school records.

Socio-demographic data, such as birth order, socio-economic status and so on, were gathered via a questionnaire that was taken home by the children for their parents to complete. However, these were not used in the subsequent analysis due to a very low response rate.

The children completed self-reports in class on perceived healthiness, amount of physical activity, handedness and sensation-seeking (using a 20-item version of the Zuckerman sensation-seeking scale, specially modified by the researchers for use in Israel).

PE teachers, trained to use a standardized protocol, gathered anthropomorphic data (height and weight) and additional trained personnel gathered data on motor ability, including agility (using the Quadrant Jump Test, jumping from one quadrant of a square to another with feet together for 30 seconds, scoring one point every time the child lands cleanly within a quadrant and 0.5 if they land on the boundary between two quadrants – this test is done twice, with a break in between, and the highest score is used for analysis), balance (using the Stork Stand Test, standing on tiptoe on one leg with the other foot of the other leg placed against the knee of the leg they are standing on, measuring time in seconds to loss of balance and using the highest score from two trials) and reaction time (using the Nelson Hand Reaction Time Test, holding a ruler in their dominant hand and letting go and catching it again, measuring the distance the ruler travels before being caught – ten trials are taken and the top and bottom three scores are discarded, with the mean of the remaining four scores recorded and used for analysis).

Injuries were measured by teachers, supervised on a weekly basis by a researcher and recorded on specially designed forms. Incentives were provided for compliance. Only injuries occurring on school premises requiring medical treatment or resulting in a limitation of usual activities were recorded. Also collected were data on the causes of the injury (type of incident), the nature of the injury (type of injury, part of body injured), severity (as indicated by the treatment required) and circumstances (location of the incident, surface, type of activity the child was engaged in and involvement of other people). These data were gathered for a complete school year.

Results

During the period of the study 73 children (3.9 per cent of the total number of participants) were injured, with nine of these (12.3 per cent of the injured) being injured twice. A total of 82 injuries were recorded, giving an injury rate of 4 per cent. More males (3.8 per cent) than females (3 per cent) and more sixth-graders (5.1 per cent) than third-graders (3.4 per cent) were injured, but these differences were not statistically significant. Most of the injuries were from falls or blows and most happened in the playground and playing fields during playtimes or PE lessons. Cuts and scrapes were the commonest injuries, but five children suffered fractures.

No significant differences in the number of injuries were found between those who perceived themselves as healthy and those who perceived themselves as less healthy or between those who were more active and those who were less active. Anthropomorphic factors were also found not to be implicated.

There was no association between injuries and handedness or between reaction time and injuries.

However, contrary to the hypothesis, those with a better ability to balance suffered significantly more injuries than those with a lower balance score. Similarly, the more agile children also experienced more injuries.

The researchers suggest that these findings can be explained by an increased degree of risk-taking on the part of those with superior motor ability (those with a more developed sense of balance and greater agility), but further research is needed to test this out.

Evaluating research into health and safety

Validity

Validity is a central concept to the effective measurement of behaviour since if a measuring instrument (be it a stopwatch or a questionnaire) does not actually measure what it is supposed to be measuring, then any conclusions drawn from data measured using that instrument are highly suspect. There, are, however, different forms of validity and it is possible for a measuring instrument to be valid in one way, but not another. For example, the Lysens *et al.* study concludes that the profiles they developed as a result of measuring physical and psychological components of young athletes accurately predicts individuals' level of risk of developing acute or over-use injuries. In other words, the profiles have predictive validity for that population. It could also be argued that they have both face validity and construct validity, given that such things as flexibility, limb speed and explosive strength are part of the profile and the data were gathered from young athletes. However, the study does not tell us if the profiles have concurrent validity, i.e. correlate with other profiles that attempt to measure the same variables.

Similarly, the Gofin *et al.* study can be said to have predictive validity, since knowing which children are more agile and have a more developed sense of balance allows us to predict that they are at an increased risk of accidental injury. Unlike the Lysens *et al.* study, however, this study does not have construct validity. Based on their theoretical understanding of the relationship between agility/balance and accidental injury, Gofin *et al.* hypothesized that the more agile, better-balanced child would suffer fewer accidental injuries, as they would be able to use their superior motor skills to prevent accidents from occurring. In fact, they found the opposite, suggesting that the underlying theory needs to be adjusted to allow for the impact of increased risk-taking by more agile, better-balanced children.

The Sherry *et al.* study also has an element of predictive validity as a relationship between distractibility and number of traffic accidents suggests that measurement of the former can be used to predict the latter, and the Raiche *et al.* study confirms the predictive validity of the Tinetti balance scale.

Ethics

In investigating health and safety there are three ethical guidelines that are of paramount importance – informed consent, confidentiality and protection of participants. In all four studies, informed consent was obtained. It is very important that this was done as the studies involved gathering personal, medically related information about the participants. This is privileged information, usually available only to the individuals (and others involved in their day-to-day lives, such as family and friends) and their medical practitioner, and so any use to be made of such data by researchers should always be cleared by the participants beforehand.

While there is little way of directly identifying the participants in three of the studies outlined above, due to the low level of information given about the participants, this is not true of the Gofin *et al.* study. They reveal that the children in the study were all the children in grades 3–6 in the eight schools in a northern Israeli city in 1995–6. Theoretically, it would be possible to track down these individuals, but no details of which individuals were injured during the course of the study, nor of which were classified as more agile etc., are given, so we can conclude that confidentiality was maintained in this study also.

Protection of participants is vital if psychology is to be able to continue to recruit participants and further develop our understanding of human behaviour. In study topics such as health and safety, it is even more important that participants are not put at an increased risk of injury simply to gather data. In none of these studies did that occur. All the data gathered about injuries related to injuries that occurred in the participants' day-to-day lives and not as a result of anything they were required to do for the study in which they were taking part.

Sampling

The use of a random sample in the Raiche *et al.* study on falling allows generalizability from the sample to the population. In other words, we can be confident that a score of 36 or less on the Tinetti balance scale is a reliable predictor of the risk of falling for those over the age of 75 years living at home. We should be cautious, however, about over-generalizing to all older people.

The more restricted cluster sampling technique used in the remaining three studies should lead to caution in generalizing the findings. In the Gofin *et al.* study, this is largely offset by the size of the sample. It is far safer to generalize conclusions drawn from data gathered from a sample of over 2000 than it is from a sample of 55 lorry drivers, as in the Sherry *et al.* study. The findings of the Lysens *et al.* study can probably safely be generalized to other young sports students, but not necessarily to sportspeople in general. It is unlikely, for instance, that such a wide variety of sporting activity is undertaken by anyone other than sports students and it could be that this frequent change of activity was implicated in the rate of injury.

Methodology

The use of correlations in three of the studies (Lysens *et al.*, Raiche *et al.*, Sherry *et al.*) means we know nothing about the causes of the injuries reported in these studies. A score of 36 or less on the Tinetti balance scale, for instance, does not mean that a person will inevitably fall over as a result. It simply means that they are at an increased risk. The cause of falling could well be due to an underlying physical condition which affects their balance and/or gait. Similarly, being a tall, endomorphic male with little static strength, great explosive strength, low muscle flexibility and a greater Q-angle of the knee than others does not mean that you will suffer overuse injuries. There could be other factors, such as the effort you put into an activity, the number of other players involved, your actual ability at the sport and so on, that contribute to the incidence of injury.

Unlike these three studies, the Gofin *et al.* study is an experiment from which cause and effect can be inferred. It is important in this study that we draw such inferences carefully. Simply being more agile and having better balance did not directly cause the increase in injuries in that group. Rather, as the authors argue, the increased agility and better balance could have led to an increase in risk-taking and thus to the children putting themselves in situations where their superior motor skills could no longer help them.

HEALTH
Health promotion

STUDY 37

Detweiler, J., Bedell, B. T., Salovey, P., Pronin, E., Rothman, A. J., 1999, 'Message framing and sunscreen use: gain-framed messages motivate beach-goers', *Health Psychology*, 18, 2, 189–96

Aim

To investigate the effectiveness of four different ways of framing messages (two positive or gain-framed and two negative or loss-framed) to persuade sunbathers to obtain and use a sunscreen.

Method

A field experiment.

Participants

217 sunbathers (165 females, 52 males), aged 18–79 years (mean age = 38.7 years), most of whom were white and of middle-income status. It was an opportunity sample gathered from a beach in southern New England, USA in August 1996. Consent was obtained and participants were given a free state lottery ticket for agreeing to complete the survey.

Procedure

Participants were given a brochure entitled 'Beach Survey 1996', which contained information about skin cancer and a number of questions. The information in the brochure was framed in one of four ways:
1) to highlight the benefits of sun-protective behaviours
2) the undesirable consequences avoided by using sun-protective behaviours
3) the benefits lost by not engaging in sun-protective behaviours
4) the undesirable consequences arising from not engaging in sun-protective behaviours.

The first two ways are positively framed and the latter two negatively framed. Participants received one of these types of information. The researchers were unaware which form of the brochure they were giving out, and so the participants were randomized to the two conditions (positive framing and negative framing).

On the front cover were some pre-manipulation questions and instructions on how to complete the survey. The pre-manipulation questions, which were answered before reading the information in the brochure, elicited information about intentions to use sunscreen that day, the sun protection factor (SPF) they intended to use (zero was recorded for those that indicated they had not intended to use any sunscreen) and asked about the risk of skin cancer; two questions, natural hair colour and skin tone, were used as an objective measure and one question, the participants' own perceptions of the risks of developing skin cancer, was used as a subjective measure.

Inside the brochure were four sets of post-manipulation questions. The first set measured their immediate emotional reaction to the information in the brochure. They were asked two questions, both rated on a 7-point Likert scale (1 = not at all anxious, 7 = extremely anxious). The first asked how anxious they felt as a result of reading the brochure. The second asked about their level of fear of developing skin cancer, prematurely aged skin or both. The mean of these two scores was calculated and used to measure the effects of negatively framed messages.

The second set of two questions focused on the participants' beliefs about the effectiveness of sun-protective behaviours. The questions asked them to consider how the likelihood of their developing skin cancer would change when they either protected themselves or did not protect themselves from the sun. Again, both were scored on a 7-point scale (1 = no change in risk, 7 = dramatic increase/decrease) and the mean of the two was used for analysis.

The third set contained two questions about how the participants thought they would feel on using or failing to use sunscreen, and two questions about how they would react to being prevented from using sunscreen (by having left it at home, for example). All these questions were also scored on a 7-point scale and the means used for analysis.

The final set focused on the participants' intentions about using sunscreen. Intentions were measured in two ways. First, they were asked questions about how often they intended to apply sunscreen over the coming month while at the beach and while engaging in day-to-day behaviour away from the beach. They were also asked about the number of times they would be applying sunscreen that day and which type of sun product they intended to use – none, tanning oil or sunscreen. If the latter, they were asked about the SPF. Responses for those using SPF greater/lesser than 15 were treated separately. A behavioural measure for intentions was taken by giving participants a voucher that could be exchanged for a free sample of SPF15 sunscreen later that day at the beach. The number of vouchers exchanged was recorded.

Results

There were no significant gender differences in the responses to any of the questions, irrespective of the type of framing.

71 per cent of those who received the positively framed information exchanged their vouchers compared with 53 per cent of those in the negatively framed message condition.

The positively framed information resulted in an increased intention to use sun-protective behaviours in those who had initially indicated that they had no intention to use sunscreen (as revealed by their responses to the pre-manipulation questions), but did not affect the intentions of those who had an initially high intention of using sunscreen. The negatively framed information did not show this effect.

STUDY 38
Chacko, M. R., Anding, R., Kozinetz, C. A., Grover, J. L., Smith, P. B., 2002, 'Neural tube defects: knowledge and preconceptional prevention practices in minority young women', *Pediatrics*, 112, 3, 536–42

| Aim | This study aimed to assess the effectiveness of a health education programme on knowledge and preventive behaviours in relation to neural tube defects (NTD) in ethnic minority young women. NTDs are birth defects occurring in the brain or spinal cord and are among the most common of all serious birth defects. The neural tube is the part of the foetus that becomes the spinal cord and brain. The two major types of NTD are anencephaly (the partial or complete absence of the baby's brain) and spina bifida (where vertebrae fail to fuse correctly, leaving an opening to the spinal cord). |

| Method | An experiment, using repeated measures design. |

| Participants | 387 low-income, adolescent and young adult women, aged 13–22 years (mean age = 18 years), from two ethnic minorities, black (286) and Hispanic (109). They were predominantly single (98 per cent of black, 83 per cent of Hispanic) and were all actively seeking help from one of three prenatal clinics in Texas, USA. Written, informed consent was obtained. (Note: originally, 22 white, one Asian and 13 other women were also recruited, but the small numbers and/or failure to return all data meant these were excluded from any analysis.) It is also worth noting that only those able to read English were included in the study. |

| Procedure | Having volunteered to take part, the participants were seen individually by an experienced health promotion nurse, who administered a questionnaire (which had been piloted for face validity on a sample of ten pregnant young women prior to the study) assessing their knowledge of NTDs, their knowledge of the preventive effects of daily multi-vitamins and folic acid and eating food rich in folates and folic acid and their actual behaviour in relation to use of multi-vitamins and eating folate/folic-acid-enriched food. The participants' responses were utilized by the nurse to give an immediate and personalized health education session on NTDs and preventive strategies. Those who indicated a willingness to take daily multi-vitamins were given a three-month supply by the nurse. The participants completed a telephone survey three months later, which utilized a different set of questions to measure the same variables as the original questionnaire. Results from the two questionnaires were then analysed. |

Variable	Pre-health education session	Post-health education session
Had knowledge of NTDs	45%	92%
Had knowledge of folic acid	52%	86%
Heard of NTD-preventive effects of multi-vitamins	50%	92%
Took multi-vitamins	9%	67%
Ate adequate amount of folate-good and/or folic-acid-enriched food	6%	37%

The study also reported that while the number of participants who took multi-vitamins increased by 58 per cent, only 9 per cent took them every day, which is the level needed for their preventive effect. Thus while the health education programme improved knowledge of the preventive effect of multi-vitamins, it did not significantly affect the adherence to medical advice in relation to this.

STUDY 39

Icard, L. D., Bourjolly, J. N., Siddiqui, N., 2003, 'Designing social marketing strategies to increase African-Americans' access to health promotion programs', *Health and Social Work*, 28, 3, 214–24

Aim

To identify which of four health promotion/communication-related factors – source, message, channel and target – had the greatest impact on the likelihood of African-Americans accessing health promotion programmes.

Method

A quasi-experimental approach using focus groups as a data collection method.

Participants

52 (five male, 47 female) low-income African-Americans, aged 26–55 years, living in a city in the north-west USA. They were divided into two focus groups, with 26 participants in each. Informed consent was obtained. Participants were paid a small sum of money for participation.

Procedure

Having been divided into two focus groups, the participants were led in a structured discussion by a trained African-American researcher. The discussion included the participants being asked questions to elicit information about:
1) the source – what type of person, such as the mayor, a minister etc., do you think should be used to disseminate information about health-related matters to the African-American community?
2) the message – what do you think a message should say in order to get African-Americans involved in improving their health?
3) the channel – what is the best way to get a message about health-related matters across to the African-American community – radio, television, newspapers etc.?
4) the target – how can the participation of African-American men in health-promoting activity be increased?
The discussions of both focus groups were tape-recorded and, in addition, a trained African-American student (one male, one female) acted as note-taker during the discussions. The data were then transcribed and their content analysed.

Results

The source – the participants reported that the source of health promotion should be credible, trustworthy, well known to the target audience and a member of that audience. They also stated, however, that the person should not have too high a profile and that credibility should not be confused with professional standing; far better to have someone with direct experience of the issue/problem/illness than a professionally qualified stranger. With regard to being trustworthy, the participants related this to the likelihood of being committed to seeing a problem through, and for this reason they were opposed to the use of politicians and members of the clergy.

The message – all participants agreed that the message should be straightforward and written in language that was familiar to the target audience (by using appropriate, non-jargon words, for example). It was also felt to be important that the message be conveyed in a tone that expressed mutual concern and not be patronizing or attempt to identify the target audience as inadequate or to blame in any way. They also stated that the message should be positively framed and promote the benefits of engaging in health-protective behaviours rather than negatively framed.

The channel – most of the participants identified one-to-one communications, leaflets and direct mailings as effective channels. Radio could be effective, if appropriate music was incorporated into the message. A problem identified with all written communications, however, was the level of literacy. Posters were seen as less effective, generally because they were not placed in appropriate locations. Places like bus stops, launderettes and other locations where people had to wait were deemed to be more appropriate than billboard hoardings. Saturation coverage was considered a good way of increasing the likelihood of the message being read, as was the use of leafleting community events.

The target – the use of sports events/broadcasts and venues where men gathered socially (clubs, barbershops etc.) were viewed as appropriate channels for African-American men. Word-of-mouth was also seen as an important channel for this group. In other words, use the channels that are best suited to the target audience. They also pointed out that it was a mistake to over-generalize the nature of the target group and that methods used to target sub-groups, such as single fathers, middle-aged men, prisoners, absent fathers and so on, should be appropriate to that group.

STUDY 40

Oh, H., Seo, W., 2003, 'Decreasing pain and depression in a health promotion program for people with rheumatoid arthritis', *Journal of Nursing Scholarship*, 35, 2, 127–33

Aim

To investigate the effect of a health promotion programme on the pain, depression and functional disability experienced by people with rheumatoid arthritis.

Method

A field experiment.

Participants

36 out-patients (31 female, five male), with a mean age of 48 years (SD = 7.5), who were regular attendees at a rheumatoid arthritis clinic in South Korea. 18 of them volunteered for the study and were allocated to the experimental condition. The other 18 (the control group) were an opportunity sample from the remainder of the clinic's out-patients, none of whom had volunteered to take part in this study. They were promised access to the health promotion programme at a later date. None of the patients had participated in a health promotion programme before.

Procedure

At the outset of the study, the three variables – pain, depression and functional disability – were measured in both groups.

Pain was measured on a four-item scale. The first item was a pictorial scale in which the participants had to select one of seven facial images that matched their current level of pain. The second and third items were visual analogue scales and measured the current level of pain and the average level of pain over the previous three days. The fourth item was a self-report on the average number of hours of pain experienced over the previous three days. All these items had been tested previously for reliability and validity.

Depression was measured with the Centre for Epidemiological Studies Depression Scale (CES-D), which had been translated into Korean in 1992 and was pre-tested on a similar group of patients for reliability and validity.

A 26-item Likert-type scale was used to measure functional disability. This scale was primarily designed to assess the extent of difficulty experienced in performing such activities of daily living as bathing, walking, going up or down stairs, gripping and so on.

Following this baseline assessment, the experimental group attended a series of two-hour health promotion sessions, once a week for seven weeks, in a room in the out-patients' clinic. During the sessions the following methods were used: group discussions, lectures, demonstrations, role-playing, contracts, weekly feedback and diaries to monitor compliance. The control group, of course, was not exposed to the health promotion sessions.

At the end of the seven-week period, all the participants were again tested for their level of pain, depression and functional disability.

Results

The results showed that the participants who underwent the health promotion programme reported a subsequent lower level of pain and depression than the control group. There was no significant difference between the groups, however, in the levels of functional disability reported.

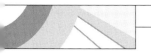

Evaluating research into health promotion

Ethnocentrism

Ethnocentrism is the term used to describe the process whereby we make assumptions about the behaviour, thought processes and so on of people from other cultures, based on the norms and standards of our own culture. With regard to health promotion, making the assumption that what works for one group of people will work for a different group is dangerous – the consequences could be continued ill health or continued avoidance of health-promoting behaviours for the second group. A good example of taking ethnocentrism into account when designing research can be found in Oh and Seo's study on pain and depression in South Korean people with rheumatoid arthritis. Instead of simply using the standard English version of the CES-D to measure depression, the researchers not only used a translated version, but also ensured that it was reliable and valid for their sample. The same cannot be said for the Chako *et al.* study on neural tube defects. Instead of amending their measuring instruments to meet the characteristics of one of their target populations (Hispanics), they chose to exclude any non-English-speaking women from being participants. This means, of course, that it is difficult to generalize from this study to any sort of wider population.

Reliability and validity

In conducting research into health promotion, it is vital to ensure that any changes in health behaviours resulting from the implementation of health promotion techniques are measured reliably and validly. The Oh and Seo study is an excellent example of ensuring that reliable and valid measuring instruments are used. They did this either by choosing instruments that were already known to be reliable and valid (the facial scale and the visual analogue scales) or by pre-testing them for reliability and validity on a sample similar to their participants (the CES-D). The level of reliability and validity in the other three studies is somewhat lower. We can assume that the questions asked in the questionnaires used in the Detweiler *et al.* study (message framing) and the Chacko *et al.* study (NTDs) have face validity, but we cannot go further than this. Similarly, the use of focus groups, with their structured discussions, in the Icard *et al.* study (social marketing strategies), suggests that the questions asked had face validity, but we cannot draw any other conclusions about other types of validity in relation to this study.

Perspectives

The most important perspective or approach that relates to research into health promotion is the cognitive perspective. This approach to human behaviour contains a number of basic assumptions. First, it assumes that human beings are not simply passive receivers of stimuli; rather we actively process and transform the information that our senses provide us with. This assumption can be directly related to the Detweiler *et al.* and Oh and Seo studies, as they both ask participants to assess a level of risk/pain. Not only do the participants have to process the question correctly, but they also have to transform a verbal response into a non-verbal one that matches the measuring instruments used. Another major assumption of the cognitive approach is that human beings are logical, rational creatures, whose behaviour is governed by the outcomes of logical, rational thought. If this were so, then we would have expected 100 per cent of the participants in the Chacko *et al.* study to have taken daily multi-vitamins and eaten an adequate amount of folate-good and/or folic-acid-enriched food after having had the benefits explained to them in the health promotion sessions, rather than the 67 per cent and 37 per cent respectively that the results showed. Similarly, we could have expected a 100 per cent uptake in the free sunscreen that was being offered in the Detweiler *et al.* study. That we did not can perhaps best be explained by another psychological perspective, humanistic psychology. While accepting the idea that we are active information processors, this approach also argues that we have free will and are not slaves to any rule of logic. Thus while a health promotion campaign can provide us with information about the benefits and losses to be made from behaving/not behaving in certain ways and logic dictates that we should then act in accordance with the beneficial message, the humanistic approach would argue that we can, and do, simply choose not to behave in that way. Therefore, while the Chacko *et al.* study points out the benefits of daily multi-vitamins, if a woman does not like taking tablets, she may well choose not to benefit from the multi-vitamins. Similarly, in the Icard *et al.* study, pertinent information may well be ignored simply because it came from the 'wrong' person. This study showed that the use of a member of the clergy as a source of health promotion information was probably counter-productive if the target audience was African-American men.

Sampling

In some ways, all these studies used appropriate samples for the aims of the study. Detweiler *et al.*, for example, surveyed beach-goers about their beliefs and behaviours related to using sunscreen rather than shoppers in a shopping mall (who may or may not have been beach-goers as well). Similarly, Chacko *et al.* used black and Hispanic pregnant women precisely because research into NTDs had not been conducted on this population before. It could also be argued, however, that using such precisely defined groups of participants limits our ability to generalize the findings of the research outside these populations.

HEALTH
Lifestyles and health behaviours

STUDY 41
Becker, H., Stuifbergen, A., 2004, 'What makes it so hard? Barriers to health promotion experienced by people with multiple sclerosis and polio', *Family and Community Health*, 27, 1, 75–86

Aim

To identify whether there are differences in perceived barriers to engaging in health-protective behaviours among individuals with different disabilities.

Method

Natural experiment.

Participants

Characteristic	Disability		
	Multiple sclerosis (MS)	Post-polio syndrome (PPS)	Polio survivors without post-polio syndrome (non-PPS)
Number	557	1730	423
Mean age (years)	52	62	62
Caucasian	93%	90%	98%
Gender (% females)	84%	70%	65%
Received some post-secondary education	48%	60%	55%
In work	29%	23%	39%
Retired	16%	39%	37%
Unable to work due to disability	35%	24%	7%

Numbers in the above table relate only to those who returned completed questionnaires, although the response rate was over 95 per cent. The participants were recruited via self-help support groups and informed consent was obtained; the Ethics Committee of the University of Texas at Austin also approved the study. On completion, all participants were sent a handwritten thank you and a $10 money order.

Procedure

A postal questionnaire was used to gather the data, with research staff available via a free phone number to clarify instructions, answer any questions or assist the participants with completing the questionnaire. Two reminders were sent to those participants who did not return their questionnaire and relevant sections were returned to those who returned incomplete questionnaires, but only after they had agreed to complete the blank sections.

The questionnaires elicited background information (gender, ethnicity, education level etc.) and also information about barriers to health-promoting activities. These were measured using the Barriers to Health Promoting Activities for Disabled Persons Scale, which required the participants to indicate the frequency with which they were prevented from taking care of their health by the 18 listed barriers. Responses were measured via a 4-point scale (1 = never, 4 = routinely).

The 18 barriers listed on the questionnaire were generated from a literature review and interviews with people with disabilities. They were then reviewed by experts and amended or added to accordingly. Items on the list included such things as fatigue, effectiveness of taking action, bad weather, availability of help, concern about safety and so on. The finalized questionnaire was tested for split-half and test/re-test reliability and found to be reliable ($r = 0.80$ and 0.75 respectively). It was also found to have construct validity in that it discriminated effectively between people with disabilities and those without.

Severity of impairment was measured using the Incapacity Status Scale. Although originally developed for sufferers of MS, it was also adapted for use by those with polio and it is known to be a reliable and valid measure of incapacity or impairment.

Other variables measured included interpersonal support and availability of financial resources. Both were measured using valid and reliable instruments.

| Results |

The main findings were that, although statistically significant differences were found between the three groups in relation to the barriers they perceived as affecting their ability to engage in health-protective behaviours, these differences were so small that they probably had few practical consequences. All three groups rated fatigue and availability of finance as the two perceived barriers that most prevented them from carrying out health-protective behaviours.

> ## STUDY 42
> Fritz, J. M., George, S. Z., 2002, 'Identifying psychosocial variables in patients with acute work-related low back pain: the importance of fear-avoidance beliefs', *Physical Therapy*, 82, 10, 973–84

Aim

To investigate the most important psychosocial factors involved in lower back pain and their use as predictors of long-term restrictions at work.

Method

A quasi-experiment.

Participants

78 people (30 female, 48 male) with work-related lower back pain of less than three weeks' duration. Their mean age was 37.4 years and they were recruited via their companies' occupational health service. 23 participants were health care professionals working directly with patients, 50 were manual workers and five had office-based jobs. Informed consent was obtained from all participants.

Procedure

At the outset of the study, all participants were given a baseline assessment by a licensed physical therapist and the following variables were measured:
1) physical impairment – this was measured by the Physical Impairment Index, a seven-item index (four items measuring range of motion, two measuring muscle force and the last measuring pain) in which each item is scored as either 0 or 1, giving a total score out of 7. This index has been tested for inter-rater reliability and construct validity.
2) pain – this was measured using an 11-point scale (0 = no pain, 10 = worst imaginable pain). This scale was not tested for reliability, but did have face validity.
3) disability – this was measured using a modified version of the Oswestry Questionnaire, a ten-item scale where each item is scored from 0 to 5 and the final score is converted to a percentage of disability. The modification for this study was the replacement of the item on sex life with one concerned with work or home-making ability. The modified Oswestry Questionnaire was tested for reliability and construct validity and was found to be as reliable and valid as the original. This also means that this modified scale has concurrent validity.
4) general health status – this was measured via the 36-item Short-Form Health Survey (SF-36), which measures eight dimensions of health (including physical function, bodily pain, mental health and vitality) on scales of 0–100. This is a valid and reliable measure of general health status for both the general public and people with lower back pain.
5) psychosocial factors – these were measured using an index comprised of seven non-organic symptoms and five non-organic signs (whose presence indicated abnormal illness behaviour), with participants indicating the presence or absence of each item, thus yielding a score of 0–12. Inter-rater reliability for this index has been established.
6) depressive symptoms – these were measured using the Centre for Epidemiological Studies Depression Scale (CES-D), a 20-item scale designed

for use by adults living at home. Each item is rated for frequency of occurrence on a scale of 0–3, thus yielding a final score of 0–60. This scale has been tested for reliability, predictive validity and construct validity.

7) participants' fear of pain and their beliefs about the need to modify their behaviour to avoid pain – this was measured via the Fear-Avoidance Beliefs Questionnaire (FABQ). This questionnaire has 16 items, scored on a scale of 0–6, seven of the items measuring beliefs related to avoiding pain at work (the work sub-scale) and four measuring beliefs about avoiding physical activity (the physical activity sub-scale). The work sub-scale has been shown to predict accurately current and future disability and work-related restrictions for people with lower back pain. Test/re-test reliability for the FABQ has also been established.

8) anxiety – this was obtained via the Beck Anxiety Index (BAI), a 21-item questionnaire with each item scored on a scale of 0–3. The BAI has good test/re-test reliability.

Following this initial assessment, the participants were randomly allocated to one of two intervention groups, which required them to attend therapy two to three times a week. The first group (37 participants) was assigned a physical therapy programme consisting of low-stress aerobic exercise (e.g. walking on a treadmill), general muscle conditioning (e.g. sit-ups) and advice to keep as active as possible, bearing in mind their pain. They were also informed by the physical therapist that their lower back pain would ease and they would return to full working duties in due course. All the participants in this group followed exactly the same exercise programme, irrespective of the signs and symptoms they identified in their initial assessment.

Participants in the second group (41 participants) were classified into one of four therapy groups, depending on the signs and symptoms they had reported:
1) manipulation and motion exercises
2) flexion and extension exercises
3) spinal stabilization exercises
4) traction.
They were reassessed at the start of every therapy session and would be moved from group to group, according to their current status. They were not given a prognosis.

After four weeks they were assessed for their fitness to return to work. Any decisions about cessation of therapy and the participants returning to work, and whether they were able to resume full functionality or have work restrictions placed on them, were made by their own occupational health staff, who were blind to the study's aims.

Results

After four weeks 21 (58 per cent) of the first group were cleared for return to work without restrictions, compared with 34 (83 per cent) of the second group, suggesting that targeted interventions are more effective than generalized ones. It was also found that those who scored highly on the work sub-scale of the FABQ at the start of the study were less likely to return to work without restrictions, irrespective of their performance on the other measures. This suggests that people's beliefs about avoiding pain at work influences their work-related health.

> ## STUDY 43
> Wilcox, S., Stefanick, M. L., 1999, 'Knowledge and perceived risk of major diseases in middle-aged and older women', *Health Psychology*, 18, 4, 346–53

| Aim | To investigate middle-aged and older women's knowledge and perceived risk of coronary heart disease (CHD) and three types of cancer (colon, breast and lung), and how knowledge and perceived risk of these illnesses varied according to age, race, education and chronic disease risk factors. |

| Method | A quasi-experiment, with data gathered via a self-report questionnaire. |

| Participants | An opportunity sample of 200 women, aged 41–95 years, living in the San Francisco Bay area, USA. Informed consent was obtained and anonymity guaranteed by the participants not being asked to divulge their name, address or any other contact details. They were recruited from a variety of settings, including health fairs, senior citizens' organizations and workplaces. |

Procedure

Women over 40 years were approached and asked to complete a questionnaire about knowledge and beliefs about CHD and types of cancer. 132 women completed the survey face-to-face and a further 131 were given stamped addressed envelopes to return the survey after completion. 68 of these were returned, giving a total sample of 200 returned surveys. Not all surveys had been fully completed and there was no opportunity to follow this up as contact details had not been asked for. This means, of course, that data from all 200 participants were not available for all measures taken.

The survey required the women to report on personal characteristics – age in years, race (due to very small numbers of women from ethnic minorities, race was dichotomized to white/non-white), marital status – and the following medical and health variables:

1) CHD risk factors were measured on a scale of 0–6, by giving a score of 0 for the absence or 1 for the presence of each of the following six items: hypertension, high cholesterol, diabetes, smoking, overweight (body/mass index was calculated on women's self-reporting of their height and weight), engagement in moderate exercise (such as brisk walking) three times a week for the past three months

2) breast cancer risk factors were measured on a scale of 0–2, by giving a score of 0 for the absence or 1 for the presence of a personal history of breast abnormalities and a family history of breast cancer

3) lung cancer risk factors were scored either as 1 or 0, depending on whether the woman was a smoker or not

4) colon cancer risk factors were scored on a scale of 0–4, by giving a score of 0 for the absence or 1 for the presence of a history of breast, ovarian and/or endometrial cancers and physical inactivity

5) whether or not the women had suffered one or more heart attacks, heart disease, angina, lung, colon or other cancers, strokes and respiratory disease

6) their current general health was rated on an 11-point Likert scale (0 = poor, 10 = excellent)

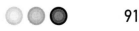

7) knowledge of causes of death (mortality knowledge) was measured by the participants being able to correctly identify which were the chief causes of death (cancer, heart disease, stroke or accidents) for two age groups (45–64 years and 65+ years) of men and women; they were also asked to identify which type of cancer (breast, cervical, colon, lung or ovarian) resulted in more deaths for women in five age groups (45–54 years, 55–64 years, 65–74 years, 75–84 years, 85+ years)

8) perceived general risk was measured by rating their responses to a question about the likelihood of a woman contracting heart disease, breast cancer, colon cancer and lung cancer sometime in her life on a 5-point Likert scale

9) perceived personal risk was also measured on a 5-point scale by asking the women the same question as above, about the same four diseases, but this time about themselves. They were also asked how worried they were about contracting these diseases, and their responses were again scored on a 5-point Likert scale

10) perceived control was measured for each of the four diseases by getting the women to rate (on a 5-point Likert scale) the likelihood of them being able to exert a degree of control over what happens should they get the disease

11) they were also asked to use a 5-point Likert scale to rate how preventable they thought each disease was

12) knowledge was measured by the participants using a 5-point Likert scale to indicate the extent to which they disagreed/agreed with statements such as 'men over 65 are far more likely to die of heart disease than women'.

Results

76 per cent of the participants correctly identified CHD as the leading cause of death for men aged 45–64 years, and 67 per cent of them correctly identified cancer as the leading cause of death for women in that same age group. These percentages fell to 59 per cent and 45 per cent respectively for correctly identifying CHD as the leading cause of death in men and women aged 65+ years. It was also found that older women were less accurate about identifying the leading cause of death in women of their own age group than those of younger age groups. Level of education was also related to mortality knowledge. The better educated the participant, the more likely she was to be correct.

With regard to perceived risk, the participants thought that they were more likely to develop CHD than any of the three cancers and had a higher risk of breast cancer and colon cancer than lung cancer. A similar pattern was found with regard to perceived control. For each of the four diseases the participants rated their own risk of contracting the disease to be significantly lower than the general level of risk.

The participants perceived CHD and lung cancer to be most preventable and colon cancer to be more preventable than breast cancer.

STUDY 44

Quine, S., Bernard, D., Booth, M., Kang, M., Usherwood, T., Alperstein, G., Bennett, D., 2003, 'Health and access issues among Australian adolescents: a rural–urban comparison', *Rural and Remote Health*, 3 (online), 245, http://rrh.deakin.edu. (accessed 14 May 2004)

Aim	To investigate whether there were differences in perceived health issues among adolescents as a result of living in a rural or urban area.

Method	A quasi-experiment, with focus groups being used to gather qualitative data.

Participants	Over 650 teenagers from rural and urban areas of New South Wales, Australia. They were all school students. The schools they attended were selected by quota sampling and the participants themselves by a form of stratified sampling. Informed consent was obtained from both the teenagers and their parents and the study was ratified by several boards of ethics.

Procedure	The participants were recruited over a period of one year (2001–2) and attended one of 81 semi-structured focus groups, with an average of eight participants in each group. 35 of the focus groups were with boys and the remainder with girls. Every group was led by the same trained researcher and items discussed at all focus groups included the participants' views on what they thought were the major health issues they faced and perceived barriers to accessing health services. Additionally, the participants raised some issues for discussion themselves and so data on these were also analysed. All the focus group proceedings were taped and then transcribed.

Results	Both urban and rural teenagers identified some common health issues, including drugs, sexual health, diet and body image, stress and depression. It was found that boys reported a higher level of perceived difficulty in seeking help for depression than girls. More rural participants than urban participants identified depression as an important health issue they had to deal with, while two health issues, youth suicide and teenage pregnancy, were almost exclusive to rural focus groups.
	Further differences between urban and rural adolescents lay in the barriers to health services they experienced. Choice of medical practitioner (availability of a female doctor, for example) was more limited for rural teenagers, and lack of confidentiality was also seen as a greater barrier to seeking medical advice and services in rural areas. Rural participants also had a lower level of medical service since there were fewer doctors and longer waiting lists than in urban areas, and financial cost was also more of a barrier for rural participants.

Evaluating research into lifestyles and health behaviours

Relationship between theory and research

In this area of psychology and health, undoubtedly you will have come into contact with theories of health behaviours, such as the Health Belief Model and Locus of Control. One way of evaluating theories is to consider whether or not there are any research findings that support the premises of the theories. The Wilcox and Stefanick study on knowledge and perceived risk is a study which investigates elements of both these theories. It shows that people do indeed make judgements about the degree of control they have over their health, and to this extent it supports the Locus of Control model and the elements of severity and susceptibility of the Health Belief Model, but it does not provide full support for either theory as it did not go on to investigate the actual behaviours of the participants in relation to their beliefs and perceptions. The Fritz and George study on lower back pain, however, does just this. This study found that participants' beliefs about avoiding pain had a direct effect on their ability to carry out unrestricted work, thus supporting the Health Belief Model's contention that beliefs can and do influence behaviour. Another aspect of the Health Belief Model that is supported by the research described above is that of the costs of acting. Both the Becker and Stuifbergen and Quine *et al.* studies consider perceived barriers to health-preventive behaviours and include among them the financial costs involved, as well as other things such as lack of confidentiality, time and so on.

Ethnocentrism

All the above studies were conducted on restricted samples, and so generalizing from them to wider populations is problematic. Indeed the issue of ethnocentrism is confounded in the Wilcox and Stefanick study in that, due to the small number of participants from the African-American, Asian-American, Native American, Hispanic or other ethnic minority cultures, they treat them as a single group – non-white. While this may make sense from a statistical/analytical point of view, it does cloud our understanding of differences in the lifestyles and health behaviours of women from these communities. It has to be said, however, that the authors acknowledge this in their paper. Additionally, part of the rationale for the Quine *et al.* study in New South Wales was that no such research into differences between the perceived barriers to health for urban and rural Australians had been carried out before, although it had been for other nationalities. In a way, then, this study was conducted to overcome the problem of ethnocentrism rather than contributing to it.

Qualitative and quantitative data

The focus groups of the Quine *et al.* study yielded rich, qualitative data, which allowed the researchers not only to identify differences in perceived barriers to health care among rural and urban teenage Australians, but also to develop some understanding of the reasons why these differences existed. This is the great strength of qualitative data. It yields far more detail than quantitative data can. It is, however, far more difficult to analyse statistically and therefore, some would argue, far less reliable than the quantitative data used in the other studies outlined above. However, it can be argued that, while the other three studies do indeed utilize quantitative measures, all they are actually doing, in using Likert scales as their main measuring instrument, is putting a numerical value to a subjective (i.e. qualitative) judgement about people's health beliefs. Thus they also have a degree of unreliability, since a score of 1 today could be a score of 2 tomorrow, and no two people interpret Likert scales in precisely the same way over a consistent period.

Ethics

While all the studies uphold the ethical guidelines of informed consent and confidentiality, both the Fritz and George study on lower back pain and, to a lesser extent, the Wilcox and Stefanick study on perception of risk among middle-aged and older women are less ethically sound when it comes to the guideline of protection of participants. While experimental protocol requires the use of a control group, was it appropriate on ethical grounds for Fritz and George to arrange for one group of their participants to receive physical therapy which was not based directly on their self-reported symptoms? The issue of protection of participants is slightly different in the Wilcox and Stefanick study, in that the questions asked could well have caused a degree of unease and anxiety in the participants, and one has to question the need for this. At the same time, however, the only way of gathering this data is probably in the way it was done. Thus the ethical question here becomes one of the ends justifying the means. The same could also be said for the Becker and Stuifbergen study, in that it may have caused some of the participants to focus on their condition more than they were ready to at that point in time.

STUDY 45
Bigatti, S. M., Cronan, T. A., 2002, 'A comparison of pain measures used with patients with fibromyalgia', *Journal of Nursing Measurement*, 10, 1, 5–13

| Aim | To test six common instruments used for measuring pain for validity, reliability and ease of use for patients with fibromyalgia syndrome. |

| Method | A quasi-experiment. |

| Participants | 602 US patients with fibromyalgia syndrome. Informed consent was obtained. |

Procedure

Every participant's pain level was measured using five common pain scales, the first three of which were sub-scales of the McGill Pain Questionnaire:
1) the Pain Rating Index (which measures the patient's perceptions of pain)
2) the Present Pain Index (which measures intensity of pain)
3) the Number of Words Chosen Index (which measures the type of pain via the selection of descriptive words; the number of words chosen is also used as a measure of pain intensity)
4) the Manual Tender Point Exam (where patients are asked to rate on a scale of 1–10 the intensity of pain felt when 4kg of pressure is applied consecutively to 18 different sites on the body)
5) a Visual Analogue Scale (where a patient makes a mark on a 10cm line, scaled from 0–100, to indicate the intensity of pain they are experiencing).

The patients were also required to complete the Arthritis Self-Efficacy Scale (which, via its three sub-scales of pain, functions and symptoms, measures perceived self-efficacy), the Fibromyalgia Impact Questionnaire (which measures physical, psychological, social and global health) and the Pittsburgh Sleep Quality Index (which measures aspects of sleep quality).

The scores on the five scales were then correlated with each other and with the other three measures.

Results

While there was a reasonably high degree of correlation between all five pain scales used, thus suggesting that they all have concurrent validity, the Visual Analogue Scale had the strongest correlation with any of the other scales. The VAS also had the strongest correlation with the Arthritis Self-Efficacy Scale, the Fibromyalgia Impact Questionnaire and the Pittsburgh Sleep Quality Index; patients reported that it was the easiest scale to complete and said they felt more comfortable using the VAS than any of the other scales.

> ## STUDY 46
> Struijs, P. A. A., Damen, P.-J., Bakker, E. W. P., Blankevoort, L., Assendelft, W. J. J., van Dijk, C. N., 2003, 'Manipulation of the wrist for management of lateral epicondylitis: a randomized pilot study', *Physical Therapy*, 83, 7, 608–17

Aim

To investigate which of two methods for managing the pain of lateral epicondylitis (tennis elbow) was more effective.

Method

An experiment.

Participants

31 participants with tennis elbow. They were recruited via referrals from ten GP surgeries in Den Haag, Netherlands. They had to have been suffering from tennis elbow for a minimum of six weeks and a maximum of six months to be included in the sample. Along with factors such as a decrease in pain over the previous two weeks, a pattern of pain that did not fit the definition of tennis elbow established by the Dutch Guidelines for GPs and shoulder and neck problems likely to enhance the tennis elbow, inability to complete a questionnaire was also used to exclude potential participants from the study. As this was to be a pilot study, only a small sample was used. Informed consent was obtained and three of the participants withdrew from the study before it was completed.

Procedure

The participants were randomly allocated to one of two treatment groups. The first group received treatment in the form of manipulation of the wrist, up to twice a week over a six-week period, with a maximum of nine treatment sessions. The particular wrist manipulation that was utilized was devised for this study and there is no existing record of it having been used to treat tennis elbow in medical literature. The second group received ultrasound, friction massage and muscle stretching and strengthening exercises, administered via nine sessions over six weeks (three in the first week, two in the second week and one in each of the remaining four weeks). This treatment had been used for this condition previously.

An independent medical practitioner administered the treatments and the researcher who collected the outcome data from the participants was blind to which treatment group they were in.

At the outset of the study, and after three and six weeks of treatment, the following measures were taken:
1) a global measure of improvement using a 6-point scale (1 = completely recovered, 6 = much worse, with a score of 1 or 2 being classed as a successful outcome)
2) the severity of the complaint, pain during examination, pain during the day and restriction of daily activities were all scored on an 11-point scale (0 = no complaints, 10 = very severe complaints)
3) pain-free grip force and maximum grip force.
4) differences between the groups were measured using unrelated t-tests or Mann Whitney U tests.

Results

There were no significant differences found between the two groups at the outset of the study on any of the measures taken.

After three weeks, 62 per cent of the group that received the manipulation was classed as having a successful outcome on the global measure of improvement scale, compared to 20 per cent of the ultrasound, friction massage and muscle stretching and strengthening exercises group. This difference disappeared after six weeks. There were no other differences between the groups.

After six weeks, the manipulation group showed a significant decrease in the amount of pain during the day compared to the other group. There were no other differences between the groups.

> **STUDY 47**
> Luffy, R., Grove, S. K., 2003, 'Examining the validity, reliability, and preference of three pediatric pain measurement tools in African-American children', *Pediatric Nursing*, 29, 1, 54–60

| **Aim** | To investigate the concurrent validity, test/re-test reliability, and African-American children's preference of three paediatric pain measurement tools. |

| **Method** | An experiment. |

| **Participants** | An opportunity sample of 100 African-American children, aged 3–18 years (mean age = 8.52 years, median = 8 years, modes = 4 and 8 years, SD = 2.55), with sickle cell anaemia. 49 per cent of the sample was female. None of the participants were in pain at the time of the study; they could all speak English; none had any known developmental problems; and the three-year-olds had to be able to arrange six blocks in size order, to indicate they understood the procedure, to be allowed to participate. Informed consent was obtained from parents and assent from the child if aged seven years or over. |

| **Procedure** | The participants were divided, for the purposes of later analysis, into age groups based on Piaget's theory of cognitive development: pre-operational (3–7 years, n = 46), concrete operational (8–12 years, n = 36) and formal operational (13–18 years, n = 18). The children were interviewed individually (although parents were usually present) and asked to recount two painful treatments/procedures they had experienced and to identify which was the most painful. They then rated each of the painful episodes on all three scales and this was repeated at the end of the session, a minimum of 15 minutes later. No painful intervention was conducted. |

The three scales used were:
1) African-American Oucher Scale (which uses either a numerical or picture scale, depending on whether the child is numerate or not)
2) Wong and Baker Faces Pain Rating Scale (in which children select a picture of a face that matches the intensity of pain)
3) Visual Analogue Scale (with the verbal anchors 'No pain' and 'pain as bad as it could possibly be' at either end).

All three scales have been previously assessed for content, concurrent and/or construct validity and reliability.

If a participant gave the highest level of pain on a measure to the incident that they had stated was most painful, then a score of 1 was awarded. If they did not do this, a score of 0 was given. The number of consistent responses (scores of 1) was totalled for each age group and then divided by the total number of participants to give a percentage validity score for that group. Only scores from the initial ratings were used for validity purposes.

Test/re-test reliability for the Oucher and Faces scale was conducted by scoring 1 if the scores given on the two separate occasions the tests were taken were identical, and 0 if they were not. A score of 1 was given if the marks made by the children on the two VAS tests were within 5mm of each other; otherwise a score of 0 was recorded.

The order in which the tests were presented was counterbalanced.

After completing the re-test, the participants were given all three scales in random order and asked to identify which one they preferred completing. That scale was then removed and the process repeated for the other two. A rank order of preference for the scales for each participant was thus established.

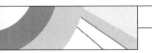

Results

Although all the participants could repeat the instructions for completing the VAS, when it came to actually doing it several had difficulty. 15 children drew horizontal rather than vertical lines, one had difficulty holding the pen and one drew flowers on the scale. These were all scored as 0. These participants were able to complete the other scales successfully and state a preference, so their data were not discarded.

There were no major problems with either of the other two scales.

Overall a test/re-test reliability level of 38 per cent for the African-American Oucher Scale, 37 per cent for the Faces Scale and 29 per cent for the VAS were found. Adjusting the scores to allow for a +/-1 variation between test and re-test scores resulted in reliability levels of 70 per cent, 67 per cent and 45 per cent respectively.

Concurrent validity for the three tests was established.

The Faces scale was preferred by 56 per cent of the population, followed by the Oucher (26 per cent) and then the VAS (18 per cent).

The results for the different age groups are shown in the table below:

Measure	3–7 year olds	8–12 year olds	13–18 year olds
Reliability	Oucher (57%)	Oucher (81%)	Faces (100%)
Validity	Faces (57%)	Oucher (83%)	Oucher/VAS (94%)
Preference	Faces	Faces	Faces

Evaluating research into pain

Ethics

When investigating pain, it is often difficult to do so without inflicting more pain on the participants. It is hard to imagine, for example, that the participants in the Struijs *et al.* study on pain management approaches to tennis elbow did not experience additional pain during their treatment. Given that the aim of the study was to try to discover which approach led to better pain management, it is possible to argue that the ends justified the means. A similar case could be made for the use of the Manual Tender Point Exam scale in the Bigatti and Cronan study on patients with fibromyalgia. The Luffy and Grove study, however, avoids this completely by deliberately excluding participants currently experiencing pain, and instead asking participants about previous painful events.

Reliability and validity

Given that two of these studies were conducted in order to investigate whether or not specific measuring instruments have reliability and validity, there would seem, on the face of it, little more to be said about these issues. However, if you delve a little deeper additional points can be made. First, although the Bigatti and Cronan and Luffy and Grove studies found their respective measures to be valid and reliable, they only established this for specific groups of people. Neither study tells us if the VAS is a reliable and valid way of measuring pain in people with developmental disorders such as autism and Down's syndrome, for example. Second, we can question the test/re-test reliability found in the Luffy and Grove study by arguing that 15 minutes between test and re-test is insufficient to ensure that the older participants had forgotten the choices they made on the scales the first time round. Thus this study may actually be measuring memory rather than pain.

Reductionism

All three studies involve some attempt to measure pain. While this is obviously important in assisting medical practitioners in their diagnosis and subsequent treatment protocols, from a more philosophical view, the use of scales to measure pain can be said to be reductionist. Pain is a physical and emotional experience which, you could argue, is not fully captured by selecting a number (as in the Oucher and Global Improvement Scales) or placing a mark on a horizontal line (as in the VAS). You could also argue that selecting a facial expression which is similar to one that you might have when in pain (as in the Faces Scale) is less reductionist than the other scales mentioned, but it could still be said that it is simply an approximation of the experience of pain that was suffered rather than a meaningful account of the reality.

Ecological validity

In its simplest form, ecological validity is concerned with the relationship between the procedures used in research and people's everyday lives. In this context, it could be said that the level of ecological validity in two of these studies was higher than in the third. In both the Struijs et al. study on pain management approaches to tennis elbow and the Bigatti and Cronan study of patients with fibromyalgia, real patients who were actually in pain at the time of the study were used. Thus it was real pain that they were measuring. In the Luffy and Grove study on African-American children, they excluded any potential participants who were in pain. While this was a sound choice for ethical reasons it does mean that they lowered the ecological validity of the study, as they then had to rely on remembrances of pain rather than measuring pain that was occurring there and then.

STUDY 48
Kessler, D. A., Lloyd, K., Lewis, G., Gray, D. P., 1999, 'Cross-sectional study of symptom attribution and recognition of depression and anxiety in primary care', *British Medical Journal*, 318, 7181, 436–46

Aim

To investigate how a patient's style of behaviour can intervene in the doctor–patient relationship to the extent that it results in misdiagnosis.

Method

A quasi-experiment utilizing a cross-sectional survey to gather data.

Participants

305 patients (225 women, 80 men), aged 16–90 years (mean age = 44 years), from a GP surgery in Bristol, consisting of eight doctors. Patients who attended both daytime and evening surgeries were included and were drawn from each of the eight doctors' panels. Informed consent was obtained and 26 patients declined taking part in the study. 24 participants failed to complete the surveys, so their data was discarded.

Procedure

Prior to their appointment with their GP, participants were asked to complete two questionnaires. The first was a 12-item general health questionnaire, which has been validated as a measure of psychological disorders. In particular, it is a valid tool for identifying the presence of depression and anxiety, where a score of three or more indicates the respondent has symptoms related to these two disorders.

The second questionnaire was the symptom interpretation questionnaire, which consists of 13 common physical symptoms, accompanied by three possible causes, one from each of three categories. Depending on the number of choices made from each category (seven or more from one category), the participants were classified as having one of three attributional styles: psychologizing, somaticizing and normalizing. Both questionnaires are self-administered.

Following this they were seen by their GPs, but told not to discuss the questionnaires with them. At the end of the surgery, the doctors, who were blind to which attributional category the patients were in, were asked to identify which patients they had noted as showing anxious and/or depressive symptoms and whether or not this was a new diagnosis.

Results

157 (52 per cent) of the participants scored three or more on the general health questionnaire, indicating the presence of depressive and/or anxious symptoms. The GPs diagnosed these symptoms in only 71 (24 per cent) patients, 57 (19 per cent) with depression and 14 (5 per cent) with anxiety.

There were 14 false positive results – patients who were diagnosed by the GP as having depressive and/or anxious symptoms, but who scored less than three on the general health questionnaire. 50 per cent of these had a previous diagnosis of depression and were undergoing treatment at the time of the study.

146 (48 per cent) of the participants chose seven or more of the normalizing causes, compared with 71 (23 per cent) who chose seven or more psychologizing causes and only 16 (5 per cent) who chose seven or more of the somaticizing explanations.

Comparisons of the doctors' diagnoses with the patients' attributional style found that doctors were far more likely to identify psychologizers as having depressive/anxious symptoms and far less likely to identify the same symptoms in normalizers. Thus the patients' way of thinking about their health (their attributional style) can affect the way they interact with their GP and, therefore, the diagnosis that is given.

STUDY 49

Schofield, M. J., Walkom, S., Sanson-Fisher, R., 1997, 'Patient-provider agreement on guidelines for preparation for breast cancer treatment', *Hospital Topics*, 75, 2, 18–27

Aim

To investigate the level of agreement between doctors and patients and nurses and patients on guidelines needed to help prepare patients for breast cancer treatment. It was hypothesized that, due to their lack of interpersonal skills training, doctors would agree less with patients on the content and need for such guidelines than would nurses.

Method

A quasi-experiment, using a postal questionnaire and telephone interview to gather data.

Participants

164 patients who had been treated for cancer in the past 18 months recruited via five breast cancer specialists in Sydney, Australia, plus 140 nurses and 64 doctors, also from the Sydney area. Informed consent was obtained from all participants.

Procedure

Each participant was sent a copy of the guidelines for preparing those with breast cancer for treatment and instructions on how to apply a rating scale to these guidelines. The guidelines were divided into two categories. The first concerned participants' attitudes to the importance of general principles about how patients should be prepared for potentially threatening medical procedures and contained 20 items about such areas as medical practitioners giving patients time to ask questions and answering them fully, avoiding the use of jargon, being sensitive to the needs of the patient and so on.

The second category contained items concerned with the specific steps that should be taken to prepare patients for such procedures, including the type of information and how it should be given before, during and after the treatment procedure. Example items from this category included asking the patient about the amount of detail they wanted to be given before the procedure and giving them an appropriate explanation of why that particular procedure had been chosen, summarizing what had been discussed, describing what was happening during the procedure and encouraging the patient to take an active part in the recovery phase, for example, by taking their own temperature.

The following 5-point rating scale was used to measure the participants' attitudes to the questionnaire items: 1 = doctors should always do this, 2 = desirable but not essential that doctors always do this, 3 = not necessary for the doctor to always do this, 4 = doctors should never do this, 5 = not sure whether doctors should always do this.

Results

Overall, there was a high level of agreement about the nature of the guidelines, with only one from the first category (about patients viewing a video of the procedure before they underwent it themselves) and one from the second category (about asking patients about their previous ways of coping) not getting agreement from the majority of the three groups of participants.

With regard to differences between the groups, doctors rated significantly fewer guidelines as important (i.e. scored them 1 or 2) than did nurses and patients. In particular, for the general principles they considered the provision of standardized written information to ensure consistency between staff, early preparation to allow time to practice for the recovery phase and the provision of additional ongoing support, for example by nurses, to be non-essentials. In relation to the specific stages of preparation, doctors regarded such items as listening to the patients' concerns and tailoring information to meet them, asking them how much detail they would like on the procedure and teaching them specific coping strategies to be less important than did both nurses and patients. These results support the experimental hypothesis.

STUDY 50
Mooney, K. M., 2001, 'Predictors of patient satisfaction in an outpatient plastic surgery clinic', *Plastic Surgical Nursing*, 21, 3, 162–4

| Aim | To investigate which elements of the patient–practitioner relationship lead to satisfied patients. |

Aim

To investigate which elements of the patient–practitioner relationship lead to satisfied patients.

Method

A survey.

Participants

An opportunity sample of 345 patients (96 per cent of those asked to participate) attending an out-patient plastic surgery clinic. Informed consent was obtained.

Procedure

Following their visit to their doctor, the participants were asked to complete the Visit Specific Patient Satisfaction Questionnaire (VSQ-9), a self-report, nine-item questionnaire that has been tested previously as a valid measure of patient–practitioner relationships and can be completed in about two minutes. The participants were required to evaluate items such as how long they waited to get an appointment, time spent waiting at the surgery before the doctor was seen, the explanation given about any procedures undergone, the technical skills (thoroughness, competence and carefulness) of the practitioner and the interpersonal skills (courtesy, sensitivity, friendliness etc.) of the practitioner on a 5-point scale ranging from poor to excellent. The responses from each participant were then transferred linearly to a 0–100 scale, with 100 corresponding to 'excellent' and 0 corresponding to 'poor'. Responses to the nine VSQ-9 items were then averaged to create a VSQ-9 score for each participant.

Results

60 per cent rated their overall level of satisfaction as excellent and 30 per cent as very good. The quality of interaction with the practitioner received the highest individual rating, while those concerned with the facilities and access to services were rated lower. The interpersonal skills of the doctor were found to contribute more to patient satisfaction than the technical skills of the doctor and were considered to be a better predictor of patient satisfaction.

STUDY 51
Smucker, D. R., Konrad, T. R., Curtis, P., Carey, T. S., 1998, 'Practitioner self-confidence and patient outcomes in acute back pain', *Archives of Family Medicine*, 7, 223–8

Aim

To investigate the extent to which practitioners' levels of self-confidence act as a predictor of outcome for patients with lower back pain.

Method

A correlation, utilizing a questionnaire to measure self-confidence and attitudes and telephone interviews to measure patients' well-being.

Participants

189 doctors and chiropractors, randomly selected from licensing databases in North Carolina, USA, who regularly treated patients for lower back pain. Informed consent was obtained.

Procedure

The medical practitioners were sent a postal questionnaire to complete. The questionnaire contained ten items such as, 'I lack the diagnostic knowledge and tools to treat someone with lower back pain', 'I know exactly what to do to treat someone with lower back pain' and 'I feel very comfortable treating people with lower back pain', which assessed their self-confidence (the first four items on the scale) and attitudes (the next four items on the scale) in dealing with patients with lower back pain. The last two items dealt with knowledge of the progression from acute to chronic low back pain and patient satisfaction with treatment. The practitioners had to use a 5-point Likert scale (1 = strongly agree, 5 = strongly disagree) to record their level of agreement with each statement. The scores for the first four items were added together to generate a self-confidence score for each practitioner and those for the next four yielded an attitude score. The last two items were treated individually.

The medical practitioners were also asked to provide contact details of any patients who came to them for treatment for lower back pain and had not yet received any treatment. Additionally, all the patients had to own a telephone and be able to speak English. A total of 1633 patients were recruited and informed consent was obtained from them. The patients were telephoned immediately after their initial visit to their practitioner, and again after two, four, eight, 12 and 24 weeks or until they had fully recovered from this episode of lower back pain. The length of time until they had returned to a level of functioning equal to that before the onset of the lower back pain was recorded.

The practitioners' self-confidence scores were then compared with the length of time taken by the patients to return to the same level of functioning as prior to the lower back pain.

Results

179 (95 per cent) of the 189 practitioners sent the questionnaire returned it, and of these 162 (86 per cent – 107 doctors, 55 chiropractors) completed all ten items.

A strong correlation was found between scores on the first four items (measuring self-confidence) and the next four items (measuring attitudes) for both doctors and chiropractors. The relationship between the item dealing with patient satisfaction and the self-confidence score was higher for the chiropractors than the doctors.

Despite differences in levels of self-confidence and attitudes among the health practitioners, there was no significant relationship for either of these factors with the length of time it took patients to recover functionality. Thus it is not possible to use a practitioner's level of self-confidence or attitude as an indicator of the speed of recovery from lower back pain.

Evaluating research into patient–practitioner relationships

Reductionism

Reductionism is an attempt to explain complex things, such as human behaviour, by breaking them down (reducing them) to a series of component parts and investigating each of these in isolation. While this approach may reveal a great deal of information about each component part, it is unlikely that it will tell us anything about the ways in which those components inter-react in everyday life. The studies outlined above all take a reductionist approach to studying the patient–practitioner relationship, to some degree. The use of numerical scales in the Smucker *et al.* and Mooney and Schofield *et al.* studies are excellent examples of this approach. Can a health practitioner's level of self-confidence, as in the Smucker *et al.* study, really be accurately described by giving it a number? Similarly, can a score of 0–100, as in the Mooney study, represent a patient's level of satisfaction? Although the Kessler *et al.* study differs from the others in that no overt scale is used, the counting up of the number of choices made from each category results in the same thing – a number representing behaviour. While these numbers allow for statistical analysis, they are, at the same time, excluding the rich detail that could be obtained by taking a more holistic approach, such as asking open-ended questions about the issues being researched.

Generalization

One of the aims of psychology is to attempt to provide explanations of the way people behave. The only way to do this entirely satisfactorily would be to investigate the motives and reasons of each and every member of the human race. Obviously this is not practicable. Therefore, psychologists study samples of people drawn from various populations, a population being a number of people with one or more pre-defined characteristics (such as age, gender, ethnicity, health status, geographical location and so on) in common. If the sample is chosen randomly from that population (i.e. if every member of that population has the potential to be part of the sample), it is theoretically possible to generalize any findings from research on that sample to that population. Thus in the Smucker *et al.* study, it is possible (because they used a random sample of doctors and chiropractors from North Carolina) to generalize the findings – that the level of practitioners' self-confidence is not related to patient recovery time – to other doctors and chiropractors in that US state. We should be cautious, however, about generalizing beyond that population. It may be, for example, that North Carolina practitioners are not very accurate at expressing their levels of self-confidence, whereas doctors and chiropractors in, say, Sunderland, are, perhaps as a consequence of having been coached in this area as part of their training. The issue of generalizing from the other three studies is even more problematic, since they all utilize very restricted opportunity or convenience samples and so the findings of each of these studies is restricted to these samples. This does not mean, however, that they are of no use outside the sample group on which the research was conducted. At the very least, the findings can provide health practitioners with information on aspects of their behaviour that may have a negative impact on the patient–practitioner relationship, which, in turn, may have a negative impact on patients' health.

Determinism and free will

The determinism/free will debate is concerned with the attribution of causes for human behaviour. Put simply, it asks the question: 'Is human behaviour the result of choices (free will) made by the person or is it the result of the person reacting to forces (either internal or external) over which the person has little or no control (determinism)?' The Kessler et al. study, for example, found that the psychologizing attribution style of a patient resulted in an increased likelihood that a doctor would diagnose depressive and/or anxious symptoms in that patient. Thus it could be argued that the doctor's diagnosing behaviour is determined, at least to some extent, by the patient's attributional style, a factor over which a doctor has little control. Obviously, the implication of this is that if doctors are aware of their patients' attributional styles, they are far less likely to be influenced by them. Similarly, the Schofield et al. study shows that the preparedness of patients for breast cancer treatment is determined, in part, by doctors' beliefs about the need to prepare patients for such procedures. Whether these beliefs are a matter of choice or determined by such things as the training doctors undergo is, of course, another question related to the determinism/free will debate.

Usefulness

While conducting research for its own sake may be a worthwhile intellectual exercise, unless that research can be utilized for the benefit of the human race we should question the value of using scant resources to conduct it. All the above studies have important implications that can benefit the service that patients receive from health practitioners. The Kessler et al. and Mooney studies, for example, suggest that the ways in which doctors are trained need to be re-examined and that knowledge of attributional styles and interpersonal skills needs to be a central part of those training programmes. Similarly, the Schofield et al. study implies that part of a doctor's training should include guidance on how to consult with patients and nurses before deciding on a course of treatment and how a patient is to be prepared for it.

STUDY 52

Vinokurov, A., Trickett, E. J., Birman, D., 2002, 'Acculturative hassles and immigrant adolescents: a life-domain assessment for Soviet Jewish refugees', *The Journal of Social Psychology*, 142, 4, 425–6

Aim	To develop and test the reliability and validity of a tool for measuring the stress experienced by Soviet Jewish refugees in adapting to life in the USA.
Method	Semi-structured interviews used to develop the acculturative hassles scale and correlations to assess it for reliability and validity.
Participants	27 Soviet Jewish adolescent immigrants living in Washington, DC or Baltimore, MD in the USA were used to develop the items for the scale. 146 Soviet Jewish adolescents (mean age = 16.13 years, SD = 1.26, 45 per cent female) from a suburban Baltimore high school, who had been living in the USA for an average of just under six years, were used for the reliability testing.
Procedure	Scale development – the 27 participants were interviewed in groups of three to five by two of the researchers, who were themselves immigrants from the former Soviet Union. The participants were asked questions about such things as their family, school and neighbourhood circumstances, how they got on with both US and Russian peers and how these factors impacted on their adaptation to life in the USA. Their answers were formulated into the Acculturative Hassles Scale. The resulting 44 items were categorized into a number of different domains (including family, school, perceived discrimination, US and Russian friends and English language) to allow different aspects of acculturation to be measured via a single questionnaire, with a 4-point Likert scale (1 = no hassle, 4 = great hassle) being used to measure the severity of the hassle. The scale was then pre-tested on a further 40 Soviet Jewish adolescents and, as a result, several items were reworded to ensure ease of understanding, five items were dropped and the school and perceived discrimination domains were combined as it became clear that most of the discrimination occurred at school. This revised 39-item inventory was then subjected to reliability and validity testing.

Reliability and validity testing of the scale – based on a literature review, the concurrent and construct validity of the newly developed scale was tested at both a global and individual domain level by correlating scores obtained on the new inventory with those obtained on a variety of other measures, including the Daily Hassles Microsystem Scale (which measured non-acculturative daily hassles), a 14-item version of the Hopkins Symptom Checklist (which measured depressive and anxious symptoms) and the 13-item shortened version of the UCLA Loneliness Scale. The inventories were administered by the researchers to the 146 Soviet Jewish |

adolescents who had been recruited for this part of the study and they were completed individually in small groups. None of them had been involved in the development of the Acculturative Hassles Scale.

Results

The study showed that the most commonly occurring and most intensely experienced hassle was perceived discrimination at school, which was characterized by the telling of anti-Russian jokes and being prohibited by teachers from speaking Russian. It was also found that girls experience more family-related acculturative hassles (such as having to act as translator for older family members and accompanying parents on various appointments) than boys.

Reliability – internal (split-half) reliability for the global scale and for each domain was found to be significant and test/re-test reliability (by having the participants repeat the inventory seven days apart) was also established.

Validity – it was found that the Acculturative Hassles Scale had construct validity as scores on this differed significantly from scores obtained on the Daily Hassles Microsystem Scale. On the other hand, the scores on the Acculturative Hassles Scale did correlate with scores on a different acculturation scale, so the former can be said to have concurrent validity. Face validity was established via the process of checking out the original 44-item inventory and changing the wording of some items and omitting five items, which had happened during the development phase. Additionally, the individual domain scales were also found to have concurrent validity.

STUDY 53

Simons, C., Aysan, F., Thompson, D., Hamarat, E., Steele, D., 2002, 'Coping resource availability and level of perceived stress as predictors of life satisfaction in a cohort of Turkish college students', *College Student Journal*, 36, 1, 129–42

Aim

To investigate the effects of perceived stress and availability of coping resources as predictors of life satisfaction in Turkish college students.

Method

Correlation.

Participants

172 participants (78 per cent female), aged 19–35 years (mean age = 21.24 years, SD = 2.01), attending a university in Izmir, Turkey. Informed consent was obtained.

Procedure

The participants were given a package containing instructions, an informed consent form and three self-administered questionnaires. All these items were in the same order in all the packages.

Perceived stress was measured by the Perceived Stress Scale (PSS), which focuses on the extent to which people perceive their life situations and circumstances as stressful. It is a 14-item inventory with items such as, 'In the last month, how often have you felt that you were on top of things?' and 'In the last month, how often have you been angered because of things that were outside of your control?' The items are rated on a 5-point Likert scale (from 'never' to 'very often').

Coping resources were measured by using the global Coping Resources Effectiveness Scale and the 12 Primary Scales (which focus on such areas as acceptance, social support, stress monitoring and health and fitness) of the Coping Resources Inventory for Stress (CRIS).

The Satisfaction With Life Scale (SWLS), a seven-item inventory, was the third questionnaire, measuring cognitive assessments of one's life. Using a 7-point Likert scale (1 = strongly disagree, 7 = strongly agree), respondents indicate the extent to which they agree or disagree with statements such as, 'In most ways my life is close to ideal' and 'If I could live my life over, I would change almost nothing'.

All three questionnaires and the other items in the packages were translated from English into Turkish by a bilingual psychologist and then back-translated into English to ensure that the items were consistent in both languages. All three instruments are known to be valid and reliable.

Results

The results showed that scores on the PSS were significantly negatively correlated with the SWLS, indicating that the higher the level of perceived stress, the less the participants were satisfied with their life.

There was a moderately strong correlation between the CRIS and the SWLS, indicating that the more available coping resources were, the more satisfied the participants were with their lives.

A regression analysis of the combined relationship between the PSS and CRIS and the SWLS showed that using the two former instruments in combination constituted a better predictor of satisfaction with life (as measured by the SWLS) than using them individually.

STUDY 54
Wager, N., Fieldman, G., Hussey, T., 2003, 'The effect on ambulatory blood pressure of working under favourably and unfavourably perceived supervisors', *Occupational and Environmental Medicine*, 60, 7, 468–75

Aim

The main aim of this study was to investigate the effects of employees' perceptions of their supervisors' interactional styles on those same employees' stress levels, as measured by ambulatory blood pressure.

Method

A quasi-experiment, with a repeated measures design. It was hypothesized that the blood pressure of participants would be higher when working under an unfavourably perceived supervisor than when working under a favourably perceived supervisor. It was also hypothesized that their blood pressure would be significantly different on a workday compared to a non-workday. A second quasi-experiment, with an independent measures design was also conducted. In this second experiment it was hypothesized that the blood pressure of those who worked under supervisors they perceived differently would be significantly different to that of workers who worked under different supervisors they had similar perceptions of.

Participants

The participants for the first experiment were selected from a pool of respondents to a previously conducted survey into favourable/unfavourable perceptions of supervisors. The criterion for inclusion was that the participants had to work under two supervisors in the same workplace on different days. Additionally, there had to be a difference of 27 points in their rating of their supervisors in the previous survey. The participants comprised 13 healthcare assistants, this occupational group having been chosen due to its low occupational status and having multiple supervisors as part of the usual work practice.

The participants from the first experiment also formed the experimental group for the second experiment. The control group for this experiment was also made up of healthcare assistants (n = 18) who had different supervisors on different days, but for this group, they had given similar ratings to their supervisors (either both favourable or both unfavourable) in the earlier survey. All the participants were aged 18–45 years.

Consent was obtained, but all participants were blind to the real aim of the study and were not informed of it after the study was over. The reason for this is that the researchers did not want the findings of the study to affect the working relationship of the healthcare assistants and their supervisors and also because the consent of the supervisors to have their ratings included in the study had not been sought.

Procedure

The participants were required to complete a supervisor interactional style inventory. This was a 47-item, self-administered questionnaire, with a 5-point Likert-scale (1 = strongly disagree, 5 = strongly agree). The items included statements such as, 'My supervisor encourages discussion before making a decision' and 'I am treated fairly by my supervisor'. On the basis of their responses to this questionnaire, which was initially completed as part of a different study, the participants were allocated to the experimental or control conditions on the basis outlined above.

Approximately three weeks later, all participants had their blood pressure taken once every 30 minutes for up to 12 hours on workdays and non-workdays. For the first experiment the workdays involved those working under both favourably and unfavourably perceived supervisors. For the second experiment the same data was used for the experimental group as for the first experiment. For the control group readings were taken for workdays working under both supervisors they had previously rated. All readings were taken using an automatic blood pressure machine and participants took the first readings on a non-workday to allow them time to get used to the machine.

Participants were also asked to record any unusual occurrences that happened to them. These were to allow the researchers to exclude data arising from unusual circumstances.

Results

In the first experiment, the participants showed higher systolic and diastolic readings when working under the unfavourably perceived supervisor than when working under the favourably perceived supervisor. Thus the experimental hypothesis was supported.

It was also found that their blood pressure was higher when at work than when taken on a non-workday and so the second experimental hypothesis was also supported.

The results of the second experiment showed that the experimental group's blood pressure was higher – 12 mm Hg (systolic) and 6 mm Hg (diastolic) – than that of the control group. This difference is not only statistically significant, and therefore supports the experimental hypothesis, but also has clinical implications, as an increase of 10 mm Hg systolic and 5 mm Hg diastolic blood pressure is associated with a 16 per cent and 38 per cent increased risk of CHD and stroke respectively.

> ## STUDY 55
> Sinha, S. P., Nayyar, P., Sinha, S. P., 2002, 'Social support and self-control as variables in attitude toward life and perceived control among older people in India', *The Journal of Social Psychology*, 142, 4, 527–41

Aim

To investigate the effects that age, perception of social support and level of self-control have on the attitude toward life and perceived control on those experiencing the crowding stress of high-density living.

Method

An experiment.

Participants

300 adults (50 per cent male), aged 60–85 years (mean age = 72.6 years, SD = 12.2), who were members of extended families and had lived in high-density housing (defined in this study as less than 170 square feet of living space per person in a household, rather than the usual method of number of rooms, due to the tremendous variation they found in number of rooms versus number of people living in a house in this city) in Agra, India for at least two years. All had at least a university education and were in a reasonable state of health and able to perform their daily activities on their own.

Procedure

Five measures were used and the researchers were examining the effects of the first three on the last two:
1) participants' age – they were divided into two groups (the Old/Old and the Young/Old), depending on whether they were above or below the mean age for the sample.
2) Self-Control Schedule (SCS) – this has four sub-scales, measuring the use of cognitions to control emotional and psychological response (e.g. thinking of good things when feeling low), the use of problem-solving strategies (e.g. being systematic in approaching a problem), the ability to delay gratification (e.g. making decisions on the basis of research rather than spontaneously) and perceived self-efficacy (e.g. boosting self-esteem through own actions). Each sub-scale is rated on a 6-point Likert scale for how characteristic/uncharacteristic each statement on the inventory is for the participant. The lower the score, the greater the degree of self-control.
3) Social Support Questionnaire (SSQ) – this questionnaire contains 27 items and measures availability of social support and satisfaction with that support. Only availability of support was measured for this study by asking participants to list all the people (with a maximum of nine per question) who could assist them in various scenarios, such as the need to talk about their problems.
4) Perceived Control Scale (PCS) – this contains 14 items focused on living circumstances (e.g. how free someone is to redecorate their room), rated on a 7-point Likert scale, was the fourth measure. The higher the score, the greater the perceived control.
5) Life Attitude Profile (LAP) – this is a 44-item measure of the existential meaning and purpose in life (i.e. 'What is life all about?' and 'Why are we

here?'). The LAP contains seven sub-scales, including life purpose, life vacuum, life control, goal seeking and death acceptance. Again, items on each sub-scale are assessed via a 7-point Likert scale (1 = strongly disagree, 7 = strongly agree). Both the PCS and the LAP have been related to increased levels of stress in other research.

Results

Age was found to have a significant effect on perceived control, with the Old/Old participants scoring lower than the Young/Old ones on the PCS, therefore perceiving that they have less control over their environment and, by extension, experiencing more stress.

Those with high self-control scored higher on the PCS than those with low self-control, as did those with high social support scores, thus indicating greater perceived control over their environment and so lower stress.

The Old/Old also scored lower on the Life Attitude Profile than did the Young/Old, and a similar pattern was found for the self-control and social support scales.

Evaluating research into stress

Ecological validity

Stress is an everyday phenomenon, with a host of cognitive, environmental and other factors playing a part in the extent to which we experience, cope with and overcome its effects. It is important, therefore, that research into stress is also set in an everyday context. This has certainly been attempted in the Vinokurov *et al.*, Simons *et al.*, Wager *et al.* and Sinha *et al.* studies, where at least some aspect of the study (development of the scale based on actual experiences of members of the target population, translating the inventories into Turkish for Turkish participants, examining differences in stress at work according to who was the supervisor and redefining high-density living to reflect local conditions, respectively) was related to the participants' everyday lives. At the same time, however, it could be argued that the wearing of a blood pressure monitor by the participants in the Wager *et al.* study slightly lowers its level of ecological validity.

Quantitative/qualitative data

You could argue that the main advantage of quantitative data is that it allows for statistical testing for significance, and any finding that is statistically significant carries greater scientific weight than those that do not. Thus all the studies above utilize numerical scales, in one way or another, to measure the behaviour of the participants and significant differences and/or relationships between variables are reported. This is of prime importance in the Vinokurov *et al.* study, in particular, since this study is concerned with developing and validating a new measuring instrument. It could be argued, however, that the quantitative data in the Sinha *et al.* study, while informing us of the effects of age etc. on perceived control and life satisfaction (and, by implication, on stress) reveal nothing about what it is like living in crowded conditions. Only qualitative data would be able to reveal such personal, detailed information.

Ethics

While none of the above studies involved inflicting harm on the participants, you could argue that having to wear a blood pressure monitor for up to 12 hours a day may have raised the blood pressure of the participants in the Wager *et al.* study, and so some minor negative impact on their health may have resulted from the study. Perhaps a more important ethical issue in relation to these studies is that of consent. With the exception of the Wager *et al.* study, informed consent was obtained from all the participants concerned. Wager *et al.* argue that, for the sake of the day-to-day relationship of their participants with the supervisors they rated as either favourable or unfavourable, it was important to keep the participants blind to the real aim of the study. It is a matter of judgement as to whether or not this claim justifies the lack of informed consent in this study.

Usefulness

The findings of each of these studies are important, not just in terms of what they reveal about the behaviour of their respective participants, but also in terms of their usefulness in helping people to deal with situations they may face in their day-to-day lives. At least two of the studies suggest the need for some sort of training for those in positions of power and authority. The Vinokurov *et al.* study on stress resulting from acculturation difficulties, for example, suggests that providing anti-prejudice training for members of the receiving community, especially school teachers, could ease the transition of adolescent refugees into a new culture. Similarly, the implications of training for supervisors to enhance the way they interact with their staff arise from the Wager *et al.* study, particularly as their interactional style could be having long-term negative effects on their staff's health status. Interestingly, both the Simons *et al.* study on Turkish students and the Sinha *et al.* study on older Indian people imply that availability of a sound support network is one of the major mitigating factors in the level of stress we experience. Thus interpersonal skills training on how to build and maintain social support could be considered for people in the situations described in these studies.

STUDY 56
Lerman, C., Caporaso, N. E., Audrain, J., Main, D., Bowman, E. D., Lockshin, B., Boyd, N. R., Shields, P. G., 1999, 'Evidence suggesting the role of specific genetic factors in cigarette smoking', *Health Psychology*, 18, 1, 14–20

Aim

To investigate the influence that two specific genotypes have on whether someone is likely to start smoking and become addicted to nicotine.

Method

A quasi-experiment.

Participants

289 smokers, who had smoked a minimum of five cigarettes a day for at least the past year and 233 non-smokers (people who had smoked less than 100 cigarettes throughout their life). The participants were aged 18–80 years (mean age = 43 years, SD = 11), 58 per cent were female and 85 per cent were Caucasian, while the remaining 15 per cent was African-American.

None of the participants had a history of cancer, were undergoing treatment for alcohol or drug dependency or had a psychological disorder that prevented them from giving informed consent. Additionally, any non-smoker whose carbon dioxide levels in exhaled air was 8ppm or greater was excluded from the sample.

The smokers were recruited via a newspaper advert for a free smoking cessation programme, and the non-smokers via a different advert seeking volunteers for a study on factors affecting smoking. All were paid $25 to cover expenses.

Procedure

All participants gave a blood sample from which their DNA was extracted. Analysis of their DNA was carried out to indicate the presence or absence of two genotypes: the dopamine transporter genotype (SLC6A3-9) and the dopamine receptor (DRD2-A2) genotype.

Every participant was also required to complete a self-report questionnaire measuring demographic features (age, gender, ethnicity etc.), smoking history (age they started smoking and length of any periods they had quit smoking for), weight, height, medication use and alcohol consumption. In addition, the Fagerstrom six-item self-report test for nicotine dependence was completed at the same time.

Results

56 per cent of non-smokers were found to have the SLC6A3-9 genotype compared to 47 per cent of smokers. This difference was significant. Among Caucasians, significantly fewer smokers than non-smokers possessed this genotype. A similar but non-significant pattern was found for African-American participants.

There was no significant difference between smokers and non-smokers of both ethnic groups in relation to the presence of the DRD2-A2 genotype.

However, 62 per cent of non-smoking Caucasian participants possessed both genotypes, compared with 46 per cent of Caucasians who smoked. A similar but not significant association was found among the African-American participants (46 per cent versus 22 per cent respectively).

It was also found that smokers who did not have the SLC6A3-9 genotype started smoking earlier (i.e. before 16 years of age) than smokers with this genotype, and they had attempted quitting less often and for shorter periods of time. There were no associations between these two variables (age of commencement of smoking and quitting history) and ethnicity, alcohol use or medication use.

There were no associations between the two genotypes and scores on the Fagerstrom six-item self-report test for nicotine dependence.

STUDY 57

Shoal, G. D., Giancola, P. R., 2001, 'Cognition, negative affectivity and substance use in adolescent boys with and without a family history of a substance use disorder', *Journal of Studies on Alcohol*, 62, 5, 675–87

Aim	

To investigate whether or not having a family history of substance abuse led to differences in adolescent boys' ability to cope with everyday problems, which, in turn, result in increased negative emotions and, consequently, the use of substances to alleviate these negative feelings.

Method	

A quasi-experiment, with self-report questionnaires being used to gather data.

Participants	

118 male teenagers with a family history of substance abuse and 158 male teenagers with no family history of substance abuse. All participants were aged 15–17 years and informed consent was obtained. Participants were recruited via substance use disorder clinics, public adverts and random selection from telephone listings. They were paid $150 for participating. Any prospective participants who had a history of psychological disorders, chronic physical disability or an IQ less than 80 were excluded from the study. Inclusion in the family history of substance abuse condition was determined by the outcome of a structured clinical interview with the boys' fathers, using DSM-III-R.

Procedure	

Each participant was given a battery of self-report questionnaires to complete. Constructive thinking was measured using the 108-item global scale of the Constructive Thinking Inventory (CTI). On this questionnaire, participants use a 5-point Likert scale (1 = definitely false, 5 = definitely true) to rate the extent to which they experience constructive and destructive automatic thoughts. The CTI has been shown to have good test/re-test and split-half reliability as well as construct validity.

Cognitive distortions were measured using the 24-item Children's Negative Cognitive Error Questionnaire (CNCEQ). This questionnaire requires participants to rate the extent to which they would or would not think in a given way (i.e. commit cognitive errors) in various situations, using a 5-point Likert scale (1 = almost exactly how I would think, 5 = not at all like I would think). The lower the score, the more cognitive errors are made. The CNCEQ has also had its reliability and validity established.

Negative emotionality or affectivity was measured using the Negative Emotionality scale of the Multidimensional Personality Questionnaire (MPQ). Individuals who score highly on this scale typically describe themselves as being in a state of worry, tension and heightened vulnerability to feelings of anger or catastrophe. This scale correlates highly with the neuroticism scale of the EPI and so has concurrent validity.

Frequency of substance use was measured via a subsection of the Drug Use Screening Inventory (DUSI) in which the participants had to indicate the number of times (using a scale of 0 = zero times, to 4 = over 20 times) they had used each of 20 different substances for each month of the previous year.

A second subsection of the DUSI was used to measure substance use problems. The participants were required to indicate the extent to which a series of 15 questions about problematic attitudes, thoughts and behaviours resulting from substance use were true to them. Both these subsections of the DUSI have had their reliability and validity established.

| Results |

The participants with a family history of substance abuse had significantly higher destructive thinking skills (and, therefore, lower constructive thinking skills), cognitive distortions, negative emotionality, substance use frequency and substance use problems than those with no family history of substance abuse.

Additionally, it was found that destructive thinking and negative emotionality correlated with both frequency of substance use and extent of substance use problems.

STUDY 58

Adams, J. B., Heath, A. J., Young, S. E., Hewitt, J. K., Corley, R. P., Stallings, M. C., 2003, 'Relationships between personality and preferred substance and motivations for use among adolescent substance abusers', *American Journal of Drug and Alcohol Abuse*, 29, 3, 691–713

Aim

To investigate the relationships between personality and preferred substance and motivations for use of those substances among adolescent substance abusers.

Method

Correlation.

Participants

200 adolescents in treatment for substance abuse and delinquency (7 per cent African-American, 39 per cent Hispanic, 48 per cent Caucasian and 6 per cent other) and 200 matched community adolescents participating in the Colorado Adolescent Substance Abuse Survey (7 per cent African-American, 40 per cent Hispanic, 50 per cent Caucasian and 3 per cent other). All participants were aged 13–19 years. Informed consent was obtained from all participants aged 18 and over. For those under 18 years, informed consent was obtained from their parents/legal guardians and assent from the participants themselves.

Procedure

All participants were given a battery of psychological and demographic assessments, conducted via a combination of structured interviews and self-report questionnaires. The participants receiving treatment were assessed at the treatment centre, while the community adolescents were assessed in their own homes.

Conduct disorder was measured via the Diagnostic Interview Schedule for Children (DISC) and substance use via the Composite International Diagnostic Interview (CIDI-SAM). The latter provides detailed information on the use of alcohol, nicotine and nine categories of illegal substances, such as solvents, hallucinogens, stimulants and sedatives, as well as marijuana, cocaine, heroin and PCP.

Personality was measured using Cloninger's Tri-dimensional Personality Questionnaire (TPQ), which assesses three independent dimensions of personality: novelty seeking (NS), harm avoidance (HA) and reward dependence (RD). The TPQ consists of 54 self-administered, true/false items, such as, 'I do things spontaneously' (NS), 'I avoid meeting strangers' (HA) and 'I work long after others give up' (RD).

Preferred substance was measured by direct questioning, although use of nicotine was inadvertently omitted.

Motivation for use was measured by asking why they chose their previously identified preferred substance over other substances.

Results

Participants who scored low on the novelty seeking (NS) scale of the TPQ tended to prefer alcohol and marijuana, whereas those high on this scale reported a wider range of preferred substances.

High NS was associated with significantly greater stimulant use and motivations focused on obtaining positive rewards, whereas low NS was associated with greater sedative use and motivations related to avoiding negative emotions or negative life experiences.

Neither of the other two scales of the TPQ was significantly correlated with substance use preference or with motivations.

In terms of differences between the two groups of participants, it was found that the treatment centre group scored more highly on the NS and HA scales of the TPQ than their community counterparts, and also displayed a wider substance use preference.

STUDY 59
Wechsler, H., Nelson, T. F., Lee, J. E., Seibring, M., Lewis, C., Keeling, R. P., 2003, 'Perception and reality: a national evaluation of social norms marketing interventions to reduce college students' heavy alcohol use', *Journal of Studies on Alcohol*, 64, 4, 484–95

| Aim | To evaluate the effectiveness of social norms marketing campaigns on the use of alcohol among students. |

| Method | A quasi-experiment. |

| Participants | Over 25,000 students and staff from 98 US colleges. As the data was gathered via an anonymous questionnaire, return of the questionnaire was taken as a proxy for consent. |

Procedure

Data were gathered from responses to the Harvard School of Public Health College Alcohol Study (CAS), which was sent to US colleges in 1997, 1999 and 2001. For this study, data from 37 colleges that used social norms marketing campaigns to attempt to reduce alcohol consumption by students were compared with data from 61 colleges that did not use such campaigns.

Social norms marketing attempts to change people's health behaviours via highlighting latent healthy norms, rather than focusing on negative aspects of health. In relation to alcohol, for example, a social norm message might be, 'Most students drink four or fewer pints when they party'. These messages are usually conveyed via posters, leaflets and so on.

Data on the students' drinking behaviour (including usual quantity and volume drunk, binge drinking and drunkenness) and their familiarity with social norms marketing messages at their schools were analysed, as were college administrators' reports about the implementation of their social norms marketing campaigns.

Results

There were no significant decreases in any of the measures of student drinking behaviour in those colleges that used social norms marketing. Indeed, on two measures – frequency of drinking and amount consumed – significant increases in these colleges were found. No such changes were found for the colleges that did not use social norms programmes.

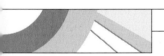

Evaluating research into substance use and abuse

Ecological validity
Substance use and abuse is a part of everyday modern living for many millions of people. It is important, therefore, that research into this area is related to the circumstances and situations of the people who engage in this behaviour. The Shoal and Giancola study on cognition and negativity concerns itself not only with the substance use of its participants, but also, via the interview of the boys' fathers, with their family circumstances, and thus could be said to have higher ecological validity than the other three studies, even though they also use self-reported data taken from

the substance use behaviour of their participants. The failure of the researchers to gather data on nicotine use in the Adams *et al.* study on the relationship between personality and substance abuse lowers the ecological validity of this particular study even further. It is possible that it may well have been the most preferred substance used by some of the participants, but the failure of the researchers to ask about it will have resulted in it not being mentioned by the participants.

Quantitative/qualitative data

In order to gather data on their participants' substance use and the other variables measured in these studies, all the researchers relied, to some extent, on the use of quantitative data. This is only to be expected, as society at large tends to use numerical values (amount, frequency etc.) to measure substance use and abuse and so, it could be argued, the use of quantitative data adds to the ecological validity of these studies. An additional strength of quantitative data is that it can be statistically analysed for significance and so lend scientific credibility to the studies' findings. A great weakness of the quantitative data gathered in these studies, however, is that it tells us nothing about the real-life experiences of using substances. This can only be fully revealed by qualitative data. For instance, Wechsler *et al.* tell us that the amount of alcohol consumed by students in colleges where they had social norms marketing programmes to reduce drinking actually increased during the course of their study. The numerical data gathered by the researchers, on its own, is incapable of explaining this. One possible explanation is that students who were not particularly interested in drinking began to feel that they were inferior to their fellows as a result of the social norms marketing campaigns and so drank more in order to fit the norm. Whether or not this explanation is valid could only be ascertained by asking the participants why their drinking had increased, something this study failed to do. The other main feature of quantitative data is that it is objective and so less open to interpretation than qualitative data. Yet all these studies, to some degree, rely on self-reports to gather the quantitative data they utilize to test out their respective hypotheses. Self-reports are, by their very nature, subjective, so we can question the reliability of the findings of all these studies. For example, it is quite possible that the adolescents in the Adams *et al.* and Shoal and Giancola studies and the students in the Wechsler *et al.* study exaggerated the amount of substances they used in order to boost their perceived standing with their peers. In addition, the use of Likert and other such scales in these studies to give objective, numerical ratings to subjective judgements can also be questioned.

Determinism and free will

The Lerman *et al.* study on genotypes and smoking, the Shoal and Giancola study on cognition, emotionality and family history and the Adams *et al.* study on personality and preferred substance use all imply that the substance use behaviours they are concerned with are, to a very large extent, the result of underlying physiological processes (genetic make-up, environmental factors and personality traits, respectively) over which we have no control. Thus they support the idea that human behaviour is deterministic. On the other hand, it could be argued that the amount students drink and whether or not they act in accordance with health promotion materials made available to them (Wechsler *et al.*) is a matter of free will. They simply choose to drink/not drink or read/ignore the health promotion material. An interactionist approach to substance use, however, would suggest that our genes and inherited personality traits may predispose us to behave in certain ways (take up smoking at an early age, drink excessively, have a preference for stimulants and so on), but these predispositions can be modified by psycho-social factors such as the behaviour of our parents and peers. This could explain different preferences for substances, as found in the Adams *et al.* study. For example, the participants simply preferred the substances that were used by their friends or family members, were more readily available etc., rather than seeking out particular substances as a result of some underlying biological drive, as the study implies.

Implications/usefulness

While conducting research for the purpose of developing our understanding is important, the ability to use the findings and conclusions of research to affect human behaviour for the benefit of the human race is perhaps even more important. The Wechsler *et al.* study, for instance, suggests that the use of social norms marketing as a means of health promotion among students does not modify their alcohol consumption, so other techniques, such as positive or gain-framed messages, should be considered. While the usefulness of this study is very obvious, the implications of the other three studies are, perhaps, more far-reaching. The Shoal and Giancola study, for example, suggests that training in constructive thinking could well lead to a reduction in substance use among adolescents. The obvious place for this to take place is in school, so this study has implications for the school curriculum as well as for health-related matters. Similarly, the Adams *et al.* study has implications beyond the immediate focus of the study. For instance, the finding that novelty seekers use more stimulants than other people suggests that if society could find ways of providing the novel experiences they want in other ways, by the development of exciting virtual realities, for example, the substance use among people with a high novelty-seeking aspect to their personality may be reduced. Perhaps the most serious implication comes from the Lerman *et al.* study. If nicotine addiction is the result of our genetic inheritance, as the study suggests, then this addiction could be removed by genetic engineering. The moral and ethical questions surrounding genetic engineering are, of course, profound, and it may be many years, if at all, before the prevention of addiction via this method is a reality.

See also...

Studies 77, 79, 104, 121, 142 and 143.

Section 3
ORGANIZATIONS

STUDY 60
Latham, G. P., Saari, L. M., 1984, 'Do people do what they say? Further studies on the situational interview', *Journal of Applied Psychology*, 69, 569–73

Aim	

1) To examine the relationship between what employees say they would do in a hypothetical job situation and what their supervisors and peers observe them doing on the job.
2) To examine the relationship between what employees say they have done in the past and what people observe them doing on the job currently.
3) To test the inter-observer reliability of the situational interview.

Method

A correlation.

Participants

29 female clerical personnel in a regional office of a major wood products company.

Procedure

Participants were interviewed using a situational interview in which questions are based on work-related critical incidents and applicants are asked to describe how they would respond. The interview included 20 situational questions and five past experience questions. The interview was assessed by a number of the employees' supervisors and peers, using an objective scoring system. Participants' work performance was measured using the Behavioral Observation Scales (BOS), a performance appraisal instrument.

Results

Significant positive correlations were found between what employees said they would do in hypothetical situations and what supervisors and peers observed them doing on the job. No significant correlations were found between what employees said they had done in the past and observations of their current performance. Significant positive correlations were found between supervisors' and peers' ratings of situational interviews. Significant positive correlations were found between supervisors' and peers' observations of employees' performance.

STUDY 61

Bartram, D., Lindley, P. A., Marshall, L., Foster, J., 1995, 'The recruitment and selection of young people by small businesses', *Journal of Occupational and Organizational Psychology*, 68, 339–58

Aim

To investigate the methods used by small businesses to select employees under the age of 20 years.

Method

An interview.

Participants

A national sample of 498 small businesses, employing a total of 5612 people. A team of about 50 interviewers.

Procedure

A highly structured face-to-face interview with employers was used to explore each organization's most recent selection of one or more young people. The recruitment and selection procedures they followed and the techniques they used were probed in detail. Data were analysed in terms of general trends and differences relating to four main variables:
1) size of business
2) geographical location
3) industry sector
4) type of occupation.

Results

The selection and recruitment procedures used by small businesses, especially those employing ten or fewer people, differ markedly from those of large organizations, being far more informal and unstructured. Among the major findings was a strong emphasis by employers on the importance of personality characteristics – such as honesty and integrity – and interest in the job. All were rated as far more important than ability, aptitude or attainment. Small businesses make more use of contacts and referral agencies than larger ones. While the traditional triad of application form, references and interview still forms the most typical pattern for selection, there is considerable variation around this. Many people do not use application forms, many do not take up references and about 10 per cent of applicants receive job offers without an interview. Initial contact between employer and applicant is more often by face-to-face meeting or telephone conversation than by letter, CV or application form. Recruitment and selection procedures used in the service sector industry, in general, were more sophisticated than those used in manufacturing. Considerable reliance seems to be placed on the 'work trial' as a substitute for selection. This may last from a few days to a few weeks.

STUDY 62
Graves, L. M., Powell, G. N., 1996, 'Sex similarity, quality of the employment interview and recruiters' evaluation of actual applicants', *Journal of Occupational and Organizational Psychology*, 69, 243–61

Aim

To examine the effect of sex similarity on interviewers' evaluations of actual applicants.

Method

A questionnaire.

Participants

400 recruiters who conducted campus interviews at a large public university in the USA during the 1990–1 academic year. 67 per cent were male and the average age was 35 years, with four years of recruiting experience. Of the applicants, 61 per cent were male, 90 per cent were seeking undergraduate degrees and 10 per cent were seeking graduate degrees.

The results are based on data from 680 interviews. In these interviews, 291 male recruiters interviewed male applicants, 166 male recruiters interviewed female applicants, 123 female recruiters interviewed male applicants and 100 female recruiters interviewed female applicants.

Procedure

Recruiters were asked to complete post-interview questionnaires concerning three of the applicants they interviewed during their campus visits. These applicants were selected randomly. Upon arrival at the campus, each recruiter received a cover letter and questionnaire. The cover letter described the study as 'an investigation of the recruitment process' and assured the recruiters of the confidentiality of their responses. The questionnaires asked recruiters to evaluate applicants on the following three measures:
1) interview quality – five items measuring recruiters' perceptions of the quality of the interview e.g. 'I got to know the applicant as a person'
2) subjective qualifications – nine items measuring factors believed to be important to recruiters e.g. communication ability, future potential, personal appearance, scholastic record, maturity
3) interview outcomes – three items measuring the outcome of the interview e.g. 'How would you evaluate this applicant's overall qualifications for the job?'
All items were scored using a 7-point rating scale.

Results

Sex similarity did not affect male recruiters' perceptions of interview quality or evaluations of applicants. Female recruiters reported better interview experiences with female applicants than male applicants and, in turn, evaluated them more favourably. Gender differences in recruiters' communication styles, social identification processes and reactions to organizational equal opportunities policies are offered as possible explanations for the disparate results for male and female recruiters.

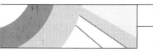

Evaluating research into selection of people for work

Interviews

All three studies described in this section involve the use of interviews. Graves and Powell examined the effects of gender on evaluations of interviews; Bartram *et al.* conducted interviews to investigate the methods used by small businesses to select employees; and Latham and Saari interviewed participants to examine whether what people say during interviews is actually put into practice in the workplace. The interview is a widely used method of research and is also one of the most common methods of selecting employees. Both as a research method and as an employment tool, the interview has advantages and disadvantages.

Interviews can vary in their structure: highly structured interviews can be little more than spoken questionnaires; semi-structured interviews are more flexible and allow the interviewee more freedom to contribute to the course of the interview; and unstructured interviews can allow for open-ended descriptions of opinions, behaviour and experience. Most interviews provide qualitative data and the more structured the interview, the easier it is to interpret and analyse the data. However, unstructured interviews will provide the richest and possibly most interesting and informative data.

A major drawback with interviews is the potential for bias, both on the part of the interviewer and the interviewee. Interviews (particularly job interviews) require the interviewer to make a subjective judgement about the interviewee and this is likely to be influenced by bias (e.g. various research studies have shown that minority ethnic group members are less likely to be successful in job interviews). Similarly, the Graves and Powell study shows that female interviewers are likely to evaluate female interviewees more favourably than male interviewees. The objectivity of interviews can be increased by pre-setting questions, having a standardized scoring or rating system and training interviewers. With regard to the interviewee, their responses are likely to be influenced by a social desirability bias, where they give answers that will portray them in the best light rather than giving honest answers. However, the study by Latham and Saari showed that what interviewees say in interviews correlates positively with what they are observed doing on the job.

Sample

The sample used in the Latham and Saari study comprised 29 female office personnel. This is a relatively small sample and the potential for individual differences between participants influencing the overall results is greater than with a larger sample. The participants are also all female, which makes the results less relevant to males. The sample in the Graves and Powell study is far larger, including 400 recruiters, generating 680 sets of interview data. However, there is a gender bias towards males in the sample – 67 per cent of the interviewers and 61 per cent of the applicants were male.

Usefulness/applications

One of the most difficult tasks of an employer is to select the best person for the job. There are a range of different methods that can be used to select employees and any research which examines the effectiveness and reliability of these methods is likely to be of use to employers. The Latham and Saari study examines the situational interview and shows that inter-rater reliability between interviewers is high and that situational interviews are accurate predictors of future job performance. Graves and Powell highlighted the potential bias in interview situations, suggesting that female interviewers are likely to favour female interviewees but that male interviewers are less prone to bias of this nature. Bartram *et al.* examined the recruitment methods used by small businesses and found marked differences between small and large businesses. Among the findings, they discovered that small business employers rated personality and interest in the job above ability, aptitude or attainment.

STUDY 63
George, J. M., 1995, 'Asymmetrical effects of rewards and punishments: the case of social loafing', *Journal of Occupational and Organizational Psychology*, 68, 327–38

| Aim | The aim of this study is to examine the effects of rewards and punishments on social loafing. The authors distinguish between different forms of rewards and punishments. Contingent rewards and punishments are those given for desirable or undesirable behaviour. Non-contingent rewards and punishments are those given irrespective of behaviour. The authors predict that contingent rewards will be negatively associated with social loafing (the more contingent rewards used, the lower the levels of social loafing) and that non-contingent punishments will be positively associated with social loafing. They propose that contingent punishment and non-contingent rewards will show no association with social loafing. |

| Method | Questionnaires. |

| Participants | 448 salespeople, working in groups of four to ten. 85 per cent of the sample was female and the average age was 41 years. The supervisors of each of the salespeople were also part of the study. |

| Procedure | All participants received questionnaires to complete in their own time and post back to the researchers. The salespeople rated their supervisors' use of contingent and non-contingent rewards and punishments on 7-point scales. Sample items include: 'My supervisor commends me when I do a better than average job' and 'My supervisor gives me special recognition when my work performance is especially good' (contingent reward scale). Supervisors rated the extent to which employees engaged in social loafing. Sample items from this scale include: 'Puts forth less effort on the job when other salespeople are around to do the work'. |

| Results | The hypotheses were confirmed. The more that contingent rewards were used, the lower the frequency of social loafing. The more that non-contingent rewards were used, the higher the frequency of social loafing. Neither contingent punishment nor non-contingent reward showed any association with social loafing. The authors conclude that positively rewarding behaviour reduces the likelihood of social loafing, but such rewards must be seen as appropriate (contingent upon behaviour). The authors conclude that punishments and rewards do not have symmetrical effects and that non-contingent responses have no positive effects on behaviour. |

STUDY 64
Drexler, J. A., Beehr, T. A., Stetz, T. A., 2001, 'Peer appraisals: differentiation of individual performance on group tasks', *Human Resource Management*, 40, 4, 333–45

| Aim | To explore the usefulness of peer appraisals. |

Method A field experiment where participants engaged in two group tasks and appraised the relative contributions of each member of the group. Participants also completed a survey measuring their satisfaction with their group and with the appraisal process.

Participants 290 students (56 per cent male, 44 per cent female) on an organizational psychology course run by a large university.

Procedure Participants worked in groups on two large projects spanning a ten-week term. The groups ranged in size, with four to seven people. Prior to the tasks the participants received training and practice in giving feedback to others. After each project was complete, each group conducted a peer evaluation of each member's contribution to the project. Each member of the group was given a rating of their contribution ranging from 80 to 120 per cent, with the instruction that the average rating for the group must be 100 per cent. Each member of the group was present while their contribution was appraised. The survey measuring satisfaction with the group and with the appraisal process was completed in the final session of the term.

Results The most interesting finding is that 43 per cent of the groups did not differentiate between the contributions of their members at all (that is, they rated each member's contribution as 100 per cent). Even when groups did differentiate, they used only five of the possible 40 percentage points available to them. Further, members of the non-differentiating groups tended to have more positive attitudes towards the group and the appraisal process than did members of differentiating groups. The authors suggest that people feel uncomfortable giving negative feedback to their peers. Interestingly, those people who were given negative feedback did not rate the appraisal process as any more negative than those not given negative feedback, which might suggest that concerns over the response to negative peer appraisal are unfounded. However, there are a number of reasons why the results of this study do not generalize to 'real' workplaces (this is discussed below).

STUDY 65
Miller, J. S., 2001, 'Self-monitoring and performance appraisal satisfaction: an exploratory field study', *Human Resource Management*, 40, 4, 321–32

Aim

To assess levels of satisfaction with performance appraisal systems and to consider the effect of self-monitoring characteristics on these levels of satisfaction. Specifically, the authors predict that those employees who are able to engage in self-appraisal, peer appraisal and upward appraisal will report higher levels of satisfaction with the appraisal process.

Method

A correlational study using a range of psychometric and survey methods.

Participants

79 project team members working in 12 teams and the 12 team leaders. These were from five different US organizations. 66 per cent of the sample was male and the mean age was 41 years.

Procedure

Appraisal satisfaction was measured by an eight-item scale developed by Harris. Examples of these items include: 'My most recent performance rating represents a fair and accurate picture of my job performance', 'The goals I aim to achieve are clear' and 'The most important parts of my job are emphasized in my performance appraisal'. These were rated on a 5-point scale (1 = strongly disagree, 5 = strongly agree).

Team members also rated their own performance, the performance of their team leaders and the performance of their peers. Team leaders rated their own performance and the performance of their team members. This was also an eight-item scale, rated on a scale of 1–5. Example items include: 'Shows a willingness to learn and improve', 'Becomes involved and participates in employee meetings' and 'Performs high quality work'. Team members were also asked whether they normally had the opportunity to appraise themselves, their peers or their team leader.

Self-monitoring was measured using an established 18-item true/false measure designed by Snyder and Gangested. This measures the extent to which individuals monitor their behaviour in response to external/social cues.

Results

Having the opportunity to rate oneself or one's team leader was positively associated with satisfaction with the appraisal system. Having the opportunity to engage in self-appraisal and upward appraisal was highly valued. However, having the opportunity to appraise one's peers or have one's peers appraise oneself did not affect satisfaction in the appraisal process and was not highly valued. The self-monitoring variable did affect satisfaction, with low self-monitors being more satisfied with appraisal than high self-monitors. This would fit with the notion that high self-monitors have a preference for career mobility and tend to have weaker attachments to co-workers. This might explain their tendency to devalue feedback from others. It certainly highlights the importance of individual characteristics when considering responses to appraisal processes (this is discussed below).

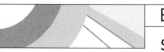

Evaluating research into human resource practices

Strengths and weaknesses of methods

All the research reported in this section used questionnaires or self-report measures. There are some obvious drawbacks to this, although there are also some strengths. In the research by George, workers were asked to rate their supervisors' use of reward and punishment and the supervisors were asked to rate the extent of social loafing on the part of the workers. These ratings are likely to be influenced by a number of factors: whether the individual likes the person they are rating; how concerned they are that the person they are rating will see their ratings; and their own subjective feelings about reward and punishment. Although the author claims to have found a correlation between use of contingent reward and social loafing, the more accurate conclusion would be that they have identified a correlation between perceived use of contingent reward and perceived levels of social loafing. It is probable that the use of an alternative method, such as observation (by an unbiased observer), would reveal different results. Similar issues may also affect the validity of the measures in the other two studies. The students in Drexler *et al.*'s research may not have wanted to appear negative about a process initiated by their lecturer and there may also be issues of ecological validity in this study, which are discussed below. Finally, there may have been other factors influencing the responses given by the workers in the study by Miller.

Ecological validity

The research by Drexler *et al.* was conducted on students as part of their course assignments, whereas the research by Miller was conducted with employees who were actually involved in appraisal processes as part of their employment. Asking students to appraise each other's performance may not give the same results as asking employees how they feel about the same process. The students would have known each other for three years of their course, would never have been asked to appraise each other before and may have felt very uncomfortable doing this. This may explain the very small differentiation that was found in this study. The studies by Miller and George were conducted with workers who rated their feelings about their work and this would give these pieces of research higher ecological validity.

Generalization

Most research in organizational psychology investigates real organizations. This obviously gives the research a high level of application to real life and will often generate a number of useful suggestions for improving work conditions etc. In many ways, such research could be regarded as case studies. This has obvious implications for the generalizability of the research. It could be argued that George's research does generalize to many other situations as it examines a basic factor affecting work. On the other hand, the research by Miller may only apply to the appraisal process as used in the five organizations included in the study. Note that this research does use more than one organization, which obviously increases its generalizability to some extent. Finally, generalizing from Drexler *et al.*'s study is difficult as it only really tells you how students feel about peer appraisals of coursework projects and it may not tell us anything about how workers feel about peer appraisals of their day-to-day work.

Usefulness

The research described in this section has many useful applications. The research by George supports the notion that reward is more effective than punishment. However, to be effective, rewards must be contingent on behaviour, that is, it must be clear what the reward is being given for. Giving rewards indiscriminately does not make people work harder and may actually increase social loafing. This is an argument that has been put forward by behaviourists for many years and has been well supported by research. From this, it might be suggested that very explicit systems of rewards (bonuses etc.) would be highly effective in reducing social loafing. Both the research studies into appraisal conclude that peer appraisal is problematic. Perhaps it could be suggested that a great deal more research is required before the widespread introduction of systems that require workers to assess the performance of their peers. It is possible that not only is peer appraisal unlikely to be accurate (for reasons discussed already), but also that it might contribute to breakdowns in worker relationships and increased dissatisfaction with jobs. However, the study by Miller suggests that self-appraisal and upward appraisal are both highly valued by workers and perhaps these processes should be introduced more widely.

STUDY 66
Senior, B., 1997, 'Team roles and team performance: is there "really" a link?', *Journal of Occupational and Organizational Psychology*, 70, 241–58

Aim	To examine Belbin's Team Role Theories and investigate the claims that high team performance is associated with teams which are balanced in terms of the team roles represented among team members.
Method	A correlational analysis.
Participants	The sample comprised 67 members of 11 management teams, each comprising four to nine members from both public and private sectors.
Procedure	Team members' roles were identified using Belbin's nine-role version of the Self-Perception Inventory, in conjunction with observation sheets from at least four colleagues who knew the member well. Team role balance was then measured by analysing each team's individual members' roles to produce a Team Role Combinations Report. Predictions of team performance were then made based on this report.

Team performance was measured using a complex repertory grid technique. A repertory grid was developed for each team, by its members. Members were interviewed individually and contributed to generating the constructs which define team performance for their team; they were then asked to rate their team on these constructs to obtain a measure of its performance. Hence each team set its own performance criteria and rated its own performance accordingly. Prediction of performance based on team role balance was then correlated with actual team performance measured by repertory grid.

Results — The actual performance of four out of 11 teams confirmed the predicted performance. The prediction for six of the remaining seven teams were within one point of the actual performance on the 5-point scale used. Only one team showed a two-point difference. A positive correlation was found between the rank order of the teams according to their predicted performance and the rank ordering of teams according to their actual performance. These findings give some support to Belbin's Team Role Theories, which associate team balance with team performance.

STUDY 67

Aronson, E., Bridgeman, D., 1979, 'Jigsaw groups and the desegregated classroom: in pursuit of common goals', *Personality and Social Psychology Bulletin*, 5, 438–66

Aim

To describe and evaluate the jigsaw group technique and examine evidence from several studies relating to the effectiveness of jigsaw groups.

Method

A review article.

Procedure

The broad background for Aronson and Bridgeman's article was the desegregation of schools in the USA in 1954. The case for desegregation included the fact that segregation sustained inter-racial prejudice and had negative effects on the self-esteem of minority groups. However, a review of relevant studies by Stephan over 20 years later (1978) found that none of the studies showed any significant increase in self-esteem among minority groups since desegregation and that a quarter of the studies showed a significant decrease. Aronson and Bridgeman's review article asks what went wrong and suggests that desegregation alone is not enough and that active strategies are needed to reduce prejudice and improve self-esteem in minority groups.

The paper describes and evaluates such a strategy known as the jigsaw group technique, which involves children working in groups of six, where they each have one-sixth of the material about a subject being taught. The children are required to share their information with each other in order to understand the whole topic, that is, they have to fit the information together like a jigsaw. During this task each child spends some time as the 'expert' and some time listening to their peers. They have equal importance and are dependent upon each other.

Aronson and Bridgeman reviewed research into the use of jigsaw techniques, including studies by Blaney *et al.* (1977), Geffner (1978) and Lucker *et al.* (1977).

Results

Blaney *et al.* found that children who had been taught using a jigsaw technique for six weeks showed significant increases in self-esteem and in their liking for their group mates. Geffner found that negative stereotypes of ethnic groups decreased following a jigsaw group programme. Lucker *et al.* found that ethnic minority children taught in ethnically mixed jigsaw groups demonstrated gains in academic performance.

Aronson and Bridgeman suggest three reasons why these studies show such favourable results:
1) increased active participation in lessons
2) interdependency, encouraging equal status contact
3) empathetic role taking – being able to see and understand things from another person's perspective.

STUDY 68
Asch, S. E., 1955, 'Opinions and social pressure', *Scientific American*, 193, 31–5

| Aim | To investigate social conformity and examine the circumstances under which people are most likely to conform. |

Aim
To investigate social conformity and examine the circumstances under which people are most likely to conform.

Method
A laboratory experiment.

Participants
123 male US college students.

Procedure
Participants were told they were participating in a 'psychology experiment in visual judgement' and that they would be comparing the length of lines. They were shown two white cards. On the first was a vertical black line and on the other were three vertical black lines of various lengths, one of which was the same length as the line on the first card. The participants were shown the first card, then asked to choose the line on the second card that was the same length as that on the first card.

The study took place in a classroom with a group of seven to nine students sitting in a line. The participant was led to believe that all these students were fellow participants, but in fact, all were confederates of the experimenter. The last in the line was the only true participant. Each of the students was asked to give their judgement out loud, according to their position in the line, so that the participant was always the last. On 12 out of the 18 trials the confederates were instructed to give unanimous incorrect answers. The experimenters then observed and recorded the response of the participant to this majority opinion. Following the trials participants were interviewed and questioned about the reasons for their decisions.

Results
In 37 per cent of the trials involving incorrect answers, participants agreed with the majority. 75 per cent of participants went along with the majority at least once. There were considerable individual differences – 25 per cent never agreed with the majority whereas other participants agreed with the majority most of the time.

During the interviews, reasons given by the non-conformists included that they had confidence in their own judgement or that they believed that the majority were probably correct but that they had to 'call it as they saw it'. The conforming individuals reported that they felt they were deficient and had to cover it up by merging with the majority; some suspected that the others were simply copying the first person, but they still yielded.

Evaluating research into group behaviour in organizations

Research methods
Each of the studies described in this section uses different research methods. The Aronson and Bridgeman study is a review article, the Asch study is a laboratory experiment and the Senior study involved a correlational analysis. Each of these methods has strengths and weaknesses and it is often an advantage to use a range of different methods to study a particular topic.

The advantages of review articles are that lots of data can be examined and they bring different research studies together, allowing for contrasts and comparisons. The disadvantages are that the studies being reviewed may be flawed or that the reviewer may be biased.

Laboratory experiments allow high control over extraneous variables, making them easier to replicate and allowing for cause-and-effect relationships to be established. They have low ecological validity, however. Due to the high levels of control, the experimental setting is often very artificial and not related to real-life situations. Participants are also likely to be subject to demand characteristics.

Correlational analysis is not strictly a research method, but a means of analysing data gathered by other means. The advantage of this type of analysis is that the nature and strength of relationships between variables can be measured; however, no cause-and-effect relationships can be established.

Data

The data collected in the Senior study were quantitative, gathered by means of questionnaires and repertory grid. Such data are easily analysed and allow for comparisons to be drawn. The Asch study also gathered quantitative data in terms of the number of participants conforming. However, this study also gathered qualitative data through interviews, recording reasons given by participants for conforming or non-conforming. This gives a more comprehensive set of data, providing not only numerical data for analysis, but also qualitative descriptions of reasons given for the behaviour observed.

The Aronson and Bridgeman study included only qualitative data, providing descriptions of the jigsaw group technique and an evaluation of studies relating to the effectiveness of such techniques. Such data are rich and detailed, but are often difficult to interpret and analyse.

Usefulness/applications

Society is made up of groups, from gender or racial groups to friendship groups or sports teams. Most employed people are also likely to belong to groups in the workplace. As such, research which examines group behaviour and how to maximize the effectiveness of a group is likely to be useful. Results of the Asch study show that, when in a group situation, many people are likely to conform to the majority, even if they feel that the group is wrong. However, the study also shows that there are individual differences and that there are some people who are unlikely to conform. It is useful for employers to know that when in a group, individuals may be inhibited from giving their view and that individual decision making may be more appropriate than group decision making at times. The Aronson and Bridgeman article examines the topic of cooperative working and evaluates a technique for improving both productivity and relationships within a group. The article suggests that the jigsaw technique increased active participation, encouraged equal status and developed empathy in group members. Such techniques could be used in the workplace for team building, encouraging cooperative working and reducing group conflict. The Senior study looked at team roles and suggested that a balanced team is likely to be more successful. This has implications for the development of teams in the workplace, suggesting that time should be spent thinking about team roles and that members of teams should be selected so as to achieve a balanced team.

ORGANIZATIONS
Interpersonal communication

STUDY 69

Kessler, I., Undy, R., Heron, P., 2004, 'Employee perspectives on communication and consultation: findings from a cross-national survey', *International Journal of Human Resource Management*, 15, 3, 512–32

Aim	

To examine whether variations in communication and consultation practices between countries are reflected in employee perceptions.

Method	

A cross-cultural study. Telephone interviews.

Participants	

3575 participants. All the participants worked in private-sector companies employing more than 50 staff. The sample comprised workers from four European countries: France, Germany, Italy and the UK.

Procedure	

Participants were interviewed by telephone. The interviews were conducted by trained interviewers and managed by ITI Research Associates. The interviewers asked for an enormous amount of information and only a few important aspects of this are discussed here.

Participants were asked to rate how often they were consulted by management and how much influence they had over decisions and also how often their union representatives were consulted and how much influence they had over decisions. They were also asked to rate the importance of eight different types of information. These included corporate-level factors, such as major changes to the company; employment-level factors, such as conditions of employment; and team/individual factors, such as decisions affecting individual workers or departments. Participants rated the amount of each type of information they received and how satisfied they were with the information they received. All the above were rated on a scale of 1–5. Finally, the participants were asked about the availability and usefulness of upward and downward channels of communication.

Results	

The results reveal some differences and some similarities between the four countries. In general terms, workers in all four countries valued all types of communication and very rarely saw themselves as receiving too much information. However, most workers tended to see themselves as having a limited direct influence over important work decisions and were not very positive in their ratings of most channels of communication (most probably due to the weakening of union powers). Workers in the UK saw themselves as more 'disengaged' than workers in other countries; they felt they had little influence over decisions and appeared to be less interested in many areas of information. Overall though, the ratings of satisfaction in the UK were still quite high and the authors suggest that this is due to low expectations on the part of UK workers. The strongest contrast was with France, where workers were very positive about channels of communication and their levels of influence. However, their overall satisfaction ratings were the lowest and the suggestion is that this is due to much higher expectations in this country. The authors conclude that national institutions are likely to shape employee expectations about the nature of communication and consultation and that this, in turn, may also affect how satisfied workers are with these processes.

STUDY 70
Orpen, C., 1997, 'The interactive effects of communication quality and job involvement on managerial job satisfaction and work motivation', *The Journal of Psychology*, 131, 5, 519–22

Aim	To examine the interaction between quality of communication and job involvement on employees' levels of satisfaction and motivation.

Method	Questionnaires.

Participants	135 managers from 21 different firms in a variety of industries in the UK.

Procedure	Participants completed a number of published scales to assess each of the variables. These included:

1) quality of communication
2) job involvement
3) job satisfaction
4) job motivation.

Results	Overall the results support the hypothesis that job satisfaction and motivation are positively affected by the quality of communication. Managers who rated themselves as being more involved were more affected by the quality of communication within the workplace. The authors conclude that improving communication within firms should raise managers' motivation levels and satisfaction levels, but suggest that this effect is likely to be stronger among managers who feel highly involved in their jobs. They suggest that strategies to increase job involvement would be highly beneficial.

STUDY 71
Osterman, M. D., 2000, 'Employee e-mail surveillance', *Network World*, 4 December

| Aim | This is a brief report on the American Management Association's survey of organizational email monitoring conducted in 2000. This research does not specifically address the effectiveness of communication via email, but does raise some important issues about the use of email technology within organizations. |

Aim

This is a brief report on the American Management Association's survey of organizational email monitoring conducted in 2000. This research does not specifically address the effectiveness of communication via email, but does raise some important issues about the use of email technology within organizations.

Method

A survey.

Participants

A random sample of large organizations within the USA.

Results

Organizations dramatically increased their monitoring of employees' email messages in the three years between 1997 and 2000. In 1997, 14.9 per cent of organizations conducted such reviews, while the 2000 survey reveals that 38.1 per cent of organizations did so. This increase is described as significantly greater than any increase in monitoring other forms of communication, such as telephone conversations, voice mail, computer usage and overall telephone use. Significantly, the survey found that over 10 per cent of the companies that conduct email monitoring do not inform employees that they do so. There are obvious implications here, with the author identifying feelings of 'invasion of privacy' on the part of employees as the most important. Osterman concludes that 'e-mail monitoring will likely end up being about as controversial as employee drug testing. The early reaction is anger, followed by compromise on the extent of its use, followed by its adoption as a standard business practice'.

Evaluating research into interpersonal communication

Strengths and weaknesses of methods
The research conducted by Kessler *et al.* is cross-cultural and compares four European countries. There are obvious strengths to cross-cultural research as they highlight factors which would not be readily apparent if a single country was studied. For example, if Kessler had only asked UK workers, the results might have suggested that workers in general were satisfied with a relatively low level of communication. It is only when one compares the British and French results that the variable of 'cultural expectations' is shown to be important. Kessler *et al.*, Orpen and Osterman are also reporting research that used questionnaire/rating scale/self-report measures. It is possible that a number of factors might reduce the validity of the information collected in this way. For example, Orpen's participants may not have been totally truthful in rating one or more of the four variables. For example, they may have felt that there might have been negative repercussions to rating their levels of satisfaction and motivation as low. The use of an alternative method, such as observation, may generate different results.

Sample

Orpen used a sample of 135 managers from 21 different firms in the UK. This is a relatively small sample, although spread across a reasonable number of organizations. It is possible to question the generalizability of findings from 135 British managers to other groups. In contrast, the research by Kessler *et al.* questioned 3575 people and this clearly gives the results a much higher level of generalizability. They worked in a large range of private-sector industries in four different countries.

Ethics/ethical implications

This type of research does not raise many ethical issues, although it is possible to consider the effects of asking participants to comment on their organizations/supervisors. People may feel anxious about doing this and have concerns about the anonymity of the information. They may also feel that the research may generate significant changes within the organization and may feel let down if this does not happen. Simply asking people about these kinds of issues may raise concerns they had not been aware of before. As well as the ethical issues that need to be considered when conducting this kind of research, the ethical implications of the research also need to be discussed. Will the research have benefits for people or could it create problems? The report by Osterman raises yet another ethical issue. Should organizations be allowed to monitor employees' personal email communications? This could be argued from both sides: perhaps employees should not be sending and receiving personal emails in work time or on work computers; however, monitoring this may make employees feel threatened and less satisfied with their jobs.

Usefulness

The research described in this section highlights a number of useful findings. The relationship between cultural expectations and satisfaction with organizational communication is a significant finding. The different levels of union representation in the different countries included in Kessler *et al.*'s research have had a significant effect on worker expectation. Perhaps it could be suggested that improved union representation would improve levels of communication. It may also raise worker expectations and this may not always be seen as a good thing by management. There are clearly political sides to this complex argument. The research by Orpen shows that improved quality of communication will improve levels of job satisfaction and job motivation. This would suggest that improving communication channels would have positive effects. However, Orpen's results also show that the improvements are most significant for those managers who already feel that they are highly involved in their jobs. This would suggest that a useful strategy would be to improve quality and communication and also investigate strategies for increasing job involvement.

STUDY 72

Scandura, T. A., Graen, G. B., 1984, 'Moderating effects of initial leader–member exchange status on the effects of a leadership intervention', *Journal of Applied Psychology*, 69, 3, 428–36

Aim

The Leader–Member Exchange model (LMX) measures the perception of the amount and quality of interaction between a leader and an employee. In this study employee satisfaction and productivity scores were taken before and after a leadership intervention. It was predicted that employees with initially low perceptions of the leader–employee relationship (low LMX scores) would show the most positive response to the leadership intervention.

Method

A repeated measures field experiment (a before-and-after intervention comparison).

Participants

100 members of a large department of an unnamed government body in the midwest USA. All took part voluntarily. The majority were female, high school graduates, aged over 40 years and working full time.

Procedure

35 participants were assigned to the leadership intervention condition and the remaining 65 to the control condition. The managers of the units receiving the leadership intervention underwent six training sessions of two hours over a six-week period, covering active listening skills, exchanging expectations, exchanging resources and practice one-to-one sessions. After training, each manager spent 30–40 minutes in a one-to-one conversation with each of their employees. The goal of this was 'to increase the level of reciprocal understanding and helpfulness'.

All employees completed a Leader–Member Exchange questionnaire, measuring satisfaction with their manager. Sample items from this scale included: 'How well do you feel that your immediate supervisor understands your problems and needs?', 'How well do you feel that your immediate supervisor recognizes your potential?' and 'How would you characterize your working relationship with your immediate supervisor?'. Statements were scored on 4-point scales. Employees also completed a number of other measures of job satisfaction and productivity scores were recorded for each individual via computer records of number of cases completed. These measures were taken before and after leadership intervention.

Results

The results were as predicted. Where LMX scores were initially low, employees responded most positively to leadership intervention and increased their ratings of both support from and availability of their supervisor. Productivity and job satisfaction also increased significantly in this group. The authors note that the employees with low LMX scores were not poor performers to begin with; they had the potential to perform at higher levels but perhaps did not feel it was worth the effort.

STUDY 73

Madzar, S., 2001, 'Subordinates' information inquiry: exploring the effect of perceived leadership style and individual differences', *Journal of Occupational and Organizational Psychology*, 74, 221–32

Aim	

To test the hypothesis that subordinates will respond differently to transformational leaders than to transactional leaders. A transformational leader is one who aims to arouse the needs of followers in accordance with the leader's own goals (the result being performance beyond expectations) and is characterized by charisma, individual consideration and intellectual stimulation. Transactional leaders, in contrast, assume leader-controlled relationships. They tend to remain quiet as long as subordinates are meeting their performance standards and may use varying amounts of positive and negative reinforcement.

Method

A survey.

Participants

75 white male software engineers employed by a large US medical technology company. All the participants had very similar jobs.

Procedure

Leadership style was assessed by the employee completing a variety of rating scales. This allowed the researchers to code each manager as either a transformational or transactional leader. At the end of each day, employees also recorded the number of times they requested different types of information from their managers. This was done for 20 consecutive workdays and the types of information were categorized into social, performance and outcome information.

Results

Overall, those managers rated as transformational leaders were asked for information significantly more often than those managers rated as transactional leaders. This was particularly true for social and performance information seeking. It was also found that transformational leaders had a significantly greater effect on their subordinates' levels of proactivity.

STUDY 74

Gardiner, M., Tiggeman, M., 1999, 'Gender differences in leadership style, job stress and mental health in male- and female-dominated industries', *Journal of Occupational and Organizational Psychology*, 72, 301–15

| **Aim** | The authors suggest that women working in male-dominated industries experience pressure to alter their leadership style and that this pressure may have negative effects on their mental health. This study examines the effects of working in either a male- or female-dominated industry on the leadership style, stress levels and mental health of males and females. |

Aim

The authors suggest that women working in male-dominated industries experience pressure to alter their leadership style and that this pressure may have negative effects on their mental health. This study examines the effects of working in either a male- or female-dominated industry on the leadership style, stress levels and mental health of males and females.

Method

A survey.

Participants

60 male and 60 female managers, comprising 30 of each from male-dominated industries (which included academia, car industries, IT, accounting, management consultancies and the timber industry) and 30 of each from female-dominated industries (early childhood education, nursing and hairdressing). An industry was considered to be dominated by a particular sex if the ratio of staff was 85:15 or greater.

Procedure

Participants were initially contacted by phone and asked if they would be interested in participating in a study on leadership behaviour and health. Questionnaires were mailed to those who agreed. Participants were also asked to nominate someone of the opposite sex in a similar position to themselves at their place of work. The questionnaires generated three measures:
1) leadership behaviour (based on the Leadership Behaviour Description Questionnaire) – this identified the level of importance placed on interpersonal relationships and the level of importance placed on the structure and completion of tasks
2) job stress (based on the Survey of Work Stress Questionnaire) – this focuses on issues such as workload
3) mental ill health (based on the General Health Questionnaire) – this measures stress and stress-related illnesses.

Results

There was no difference in interpersonal orientation between male and female leaders working in male-dominated industries. However, women working in female-dominated industries were more interpersonally oriented than men. Women working in male-dominated industries reported the highest levels of pressure and experienced the worst mental health. This was particularly significant when the women adopted an interpersonal orientation. The findings strongly suggest that both gender and the gender ratio of the work environment influence leadership style, stress and mental health and the authors suggest that the findings contribute significantly to our understanding of the barriers to women working in senior management positions in male-dominated industries.

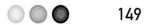

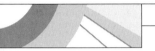

Evaluating research into leadership and management

Importance of other contributing factors

In all these studies, there may be other factors contributing to the results which have not been considered in the research. For example, in the study by Gardiner and Tiggeman, it is possible that other factors have contributed to the levels of stress and mental health problems experienced by the female participants. It may be that domestic pressures, such as childcare, or conflicts experienced between work and home responsibilities may be greater for women. It may also be possible that male-dominated industries do not respond in the same way to problems such as these. This does not detract from the findings that adopting certain management styles may affect stress/mental health, but it is likely that a number of other factors need to be considered. In the research by Scandura and Graen, there may be alternative explanations for the findings. The fact that some intervention has taken place and each employee has had a one-to-one conversation with their manager may explain the increase in scores for the intervention group. In other words, it may not be the specific leadership training that had the effect.

Strengths and weaknesses of method

The studies reported in this section have used a variety of rating scales and questionnaires to assess aspects of leadership behaviour and related variables. There are many strengths associated with this method, including the ease with which data can be collected and analysed and the fact that many of these scales have been standardized. However, people's self-reports of behaviour may be inaccurate for a number of reasons (lack of insight into their own behaviour, demand characteristics, social desirability bias and so on) and using different methods to assess leadership behaviour may reveal different results. For example, in the study by Gardiner and Tiggeman, participants rated their own leadership behaviour. If this had been conducted as an observation, with experienced observers rating the behaviour of the participants, this might have shown different patterns. In the study by Madzar, employees rated their perceptions of the leadership style of their manager and there may be a number of biases here. Employees who have poor relationships with their managers or who have been reprimanded may take advantage of this exercise to give negative feedback on the manager. Alternatively, employees may be concerned that their managers would see the ratings they give and this would invariably lead them to say nothing that might be interpreted negatively. Finally, it is also possible that employees' recordings of the frequency and type of information that was sought might be inaccurate, either because they do not record every instance or because there might be other sources of information that are not recorded. For example, feedback on some tasks may be easier to get from colleagues and this could have been taken into account. Again, suggesting an observation using trained observers might give more valid results.

Sample/generalization

There are a number of issues that could be discussed under this heading. The sample sizes are relatively similar and fairly small, which may make generalization to other groups difficult. The research by Madzar concentrated on a homogeneous group of male software engineers employed in a single US industry. While there are no doubt advantages to concentrating research in this way, it is clearly difficult to generalize the findings to other groups: females, other occupations, other industries, other countries and so on. The research by Scandura and Graen also suffers from this problem, although in this study the sample was female. In contrast, the research by Gardiner and Tiggeman used participants from a variety of occupations and compared genders. This revealed some significant gender differences and this would strengthen the argument that it would be difficult to generalize from research conducted on one gender to the other.

Usefulness

There are a number of useful applications that could be raised here. Gardiner and Tiggeman suggest that it would be counterproductive to imply that women in male-dominated industries should change their leadership orientation. However, they do suggest that women working in male-dominated industries may require training for women that would help them to deal with the problems arising from adopting particular leadership styles. Further, it could be suggested that the prevailing culture in male-dominated industries needs addressing and that women would benefit from changes in institutional practices and expectations. Scandula and Graen's research shows that it is possible to improve leadership skills and that this will have a number of positive effects. Madzar's research suggests that transformational leaders are more effective and it could be suggested that training in the skills associated with this style of leadership would enhance the effectiveness of many managers and hence the productivity of the organization.

ORGANIZATIONS
Motivation to work

STUDY 75

Yearta, S. K., Maitlis, S., Briner, R. B., 1995, 'An exploratory study of goal setting in theory and practice: a motivational technique that works?', *Journal of Occupational and Organizational Psychology*, 68, 237–52

Aim	To examine the relationship between goal difficulty, participation in the goal-setting process and goal performance in an organizational setting.
Method	A field experiment.
Participants	132 employees and 27 of their supervisors at the research centre of a large multinational company. Most of the work carried out was scientific and highly specialized and the majority of the participants possessed postgraduate degrees.

Goal setting had been implemented in the company three years prior to the study. Three goals were set for each individual, each year, as part of their annual performance appraisal review. Goals were set by job holders and their supervisors, with employees being encouraged to become as involved as possible in the goal-setting process. However, there was no formal policy regarding the degree of employee participation in this process.

The present study took place five months after employee goals had been set.

Procedure

Questionnaires were distributed to job holders and their supervisors. The job holders' questionnaire instructed respondents to indicate the extent to which they agreed or disagreed with statements relating to each of their three goals in terms of its difficulty, the degree to which they participated in setting it and their perceptions of their performance to date relating to the goal.

Supervisors were asked to complete a similar questionnaire relating to the individuals they supervised in terms of goal difficulty, job-holder participation in setting the goal and their perceptions of each employee's performance relating to the goal.

Results

Results were analysed to establish the relationship between goal difficulty and goal performance and the relationship between participation in the goal-setting process and goal performance. Based on goal-setting theory and the results of previous experimental research, high levels of goal difficulty were predicted to be associated with high goal performance. However, results of this study showed a moderate but significant negative correlation between goal difficulty and goal performance – the more difficult the goal, the lower the level of performance. Weak but significant correlations were found between supervisor and job-holder ratings of participation in goal setting and their own ratings of goal performance.

STUDY 76
Hollenbeck, J. R., Williams, C. R., Klein, H. J., 1989, 'An empirical examination of the antecedents of commitment to difficult goals', *Journal of Applied Psychology*, 74, 1, 18–23

Aim

To examine the factors that contribute to commitment to difficult goals.

Method

A field experiment.

Participants

451 undergraduate students (reduced to 190 through uncontrolled and planned attrition) enrolled on an introductory management course at a large midwestern university in the USA. Participants received a small amount of extra credit in return for their participation.

Procedure

The following hypotheses were tested:
1) commitment to difficult goals is greater when goals are made public than when they are kept private
2) commitment to difficult goals is higher under self-set goal conditions than under assignment conditions
3) commitment to difficult goals is positively related to Need to Achieve
4) commitment to difficult goals is negatively related to externality of Locus of Control.

Participants were recruited from classes during the first week of term and told that the researchers were investigating the effects of goal setting on academic performance. At the first session they completed a questionnaire that assessed Locus of Control (the extent to which we feel in personal control of events) and Need to Achieve (the extent to which we are motivated by the desire to achieve success); their permission was also sought for researchers to obtain prior Grade Point Averages (GPA) and GPAs while the study was being conducted.

Participants were assigned to different groups. They were put into either a self-set or an assigned condition and either a private or public condition, with the following characteristics:
1) self-set condition – participants selected a hard GPA goal for themselves for the next academic quarter
2) assigned condition – a hard GPA goal was assigned to participants for the next academic quarter
3) private condition – GPA goal remained confidential
4) public condition – participant's name and GPA goal was made available to the other participants in that condition and to a self-determined significant other (usually a parent or sibling).

The dependent variables included goal commitment, measured by a nine-item self-report measure designed for the experiment, and GPA performance, measured by the difference between GPA for the quarter during which the experiment took place and prior GPA.

Results	

The public goal condition resulted in higher goal commitment than the private goal condition. Goal commitment was highest for participants with an internal Locus of Control and high Need to Achieve. The relationship between Need to Achieve and goal commitment is stronger when goals are self-set rather than when they are assigned.

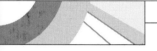

Evaluating research into motivation to work

Field experiments

Both the Hollenbeck *et al.* study and the Yearta *et al.* study use the field experiment method of research, an experimental method which involves studying participants in a natural environment but where the independent variable is manipulated by the experimenter. As a research method this has both advantages and disadvantages. The advantages include greater ecological validity, as the experiment is conducted in realistic conditions. In the Hollenbeck *et al.* study students were observed and tested as they completed an academic quarter of a management course at a US university. In the Yearta *et al.* study participants were tested in their normal work environment. The advantage of high ecological validity is that the results can be generalized more easily to everyday life situations.

However, in both studies, participants were aware that they were participating in an experiment and so demand characteristics may have influenced their behaviour. A further disadvantage of field experiments is that they are harder to control than laboratory studies; for example, in the Hollenbeck *et al.* study the researchers would have been unable to control other factors that may have contributed to participants' GPAs during the academic quarter. This lack of control makes cause-and-effect relationships more difficult to establish and replication more difficult.

Sampling

The sample used in the Hollenbeck *et al.* study comprised 451 undergraduate students who received course credits in return for participation. This is likely to be an unrepresentative sample as students are unlike the general population in many ways – they may be more familiar with setting and working towards goals, for example. The fact that they received course credits may have influenced their behaviour also, making them more helpful and cooperative towards the experimenter.

The sample in the Yearta *et al.* study comprised 132 employees and 27 supervisors at a multinational company. This is a fairly large sample, which makes individual differences between participants less likely to influence the results. However, the majority of the participants possessed postgraduate degrees and were involved in highly specialized scientific work. This makes the sample atypical of the general population and limits the groups in society to whom these results can be generalized.

Data

In both these studies the data collected were quantitative. In the Yearta *et al.* study this was by means of questionnaires and in the Hollenbeck *et al.* study both questionnaires and GPA scores were used to generate quantitative data. The advantages of this type of numerical data include the ease with which it can be analysed statistically and comparisons made between individuals and groups. However, the studies both lack descriptive or qualitative data, which may have provided more of an insight into the extent to which participants felt motivated by the goals and the reasons why they performed better under some conditions than others.

Usefulness/applications

Both these studies are useful in that they examine different ways of improving motivation. The Hollenbeck *et al.* study showed that commitment to goals was greater when the goals were self-set and when they were made public. The Yearta *et al.* study confirms that participation in goal setting leads to better performance, but also showed, contrary to previous research, that the more difficult the goal, the lower the level of performance. These studies show the value of goal setting as a motivational force and suggest conditions under which goal setting is likely to be most effective and productive. This is useful and valuable information for employers in any sector.

ORGANIZATIONS
Quality of working life

STUDY 77
Swanson, V., Power, K. G., Simpson, R. J., 1998, 'Occupational stress and family life: a comparison of male and female doctors', *Journal of Occupational and Organizational Psychology*, 71, 237–60

Aim	To investigate stress in the interface between home and work, comparing male and female doctors working in general practice and consultant specialities.

Method A questionnaire survey.

Participants A questionnaire survey was sent to 1668 doctors selected to represent all Scottish Health Boards. A sample was selected alphabetically from Health Board lists to form four approximately equal-sized gender and speciality groups. Replies were returned anonymously to maintain confidentiality. The final sample comprised 986 doctors, including 283 female GPs, 224 female consultants, 264 male GPs and 215 male consultants.

Procedure Participants completed a questionnaire, which included the following measures:
1) demographic information e.g. age, speciality, marital status
2) domestic role complexity e.g. number and age of children
3) work load i.e. average number of hours worked per week and on call
4) occupational stress measured by scales taken from the Occupational Stress Indicator (OSI)
5) home/work stress
6) job satisfaction
7) home stress
8) domestic conflict
9) domestic satisfaction.

The following hypotheses were tested:
1) females with greater 'role complexity' would be more likely to adapt working hours and domestic work hours to family demands
2) increased complexity of domestic roles will be significantly associated with increased occupational stress or decreased job satisfaction and the nature of this relationship would be more significant for females than males and more significant for doctors than consultants
3) levels of home to work (HW) stress but not work to home (WH) stress would increase with role complexity
4) females would have greater HW stress but not greater WH stress than males.

Results Increasing domestic role demands were related to stress for both female and male doctors. Increased role complexity was significantly related to WH stress for both sexes. Increased domestic role complexity was related to reduced occupational work hours for female doctors but not for males. There was no significant relationship between increased domestic role complexity and job satisfaction.

STUDY 78
Wright, T. A., Cropanzano, R., 'Emotional exhaustion as a predictor of job performance and voluntary turnover', *Journal of Applied Psychology*, 83, 3, 486–93

| Aim | To examine the relationship between emotional exhaustion and job satisfaction, voluntary turnover and job performance. The personality dispositions of positive affectivity and negative affectivity were used as control variables. |

| Method | A longitudinal study. |

| Participants | 52 social welfare workers employed by a large city on the west coast of the USA. All had completed Bachelors degrees and were employed within the same department and performed the same duties. 69 per cent were male and the mean age was 42 years. |

| Procedure | The following variables were measured at the start of the study and one year later: |

1) emotional exhaustion – using the Maslach Burn-out Inventory (a nine-item scale measuring how often one feels emotionally over-extended and exhausted by one's work)
2) job satisfaction – using a five-item scale measuring degree of satisfaction with co-workers, supervisors, promotional opportunities and pay
3) performance – assessed by the same top-ranking administration officer answering the following question: 'How would you rate this employee's performance over the last six months?' using a 5-point rating scale (1 = poor, 5 = excellent)
4) turnover – voluntary withdrawal from the organization
5) dispositional affectivity – using the Positive and Negative Affectivity Schedule (PANAS) designed to measure the personality dispositions of negative affectivity (NA – high negative emotions) and positive affectivity (PA – high positive emotions).

The following hypotheses were tested:
1) job satisfaction will be negatively related to emotional exhaustion
2) job performance will be negatively related to emotional exhaustion
3) emotional exhaustion will be positively related to subsequent voluntary employee turnover
4) NA will be positively related to emotional exhaustion; PA will be negatively related to emotional exhaustion
5) all the relationships predicted in hypotheses 1–3 will remain significant even after controlling for the effects of NA and PA.

| Results | Hypothesis 1, predicting a negative relationship between emotional exhaustion and job satisfaction, was not supported. Emotional exhaustion was negatively correlated with job performance. A positive relationship was established between emotional exhaustion and voluntary turnover. A negative relationship was established between PA and emotional exhaustion. A positive relationship was established between NA and emotional exhaustion. The relationship between emotional exhaustion and performance and also between emotional exhaustion and turnover remain significant above and beyond the effects of PA and NA. |

STUDY 79

Jones, F., Fletcher, B., 1996, 'Taking work home: a study of daily fluctuations in work stressors, effects on moods and impacts on marital partners', *Journal of Occupational and Organizational Psychology*, 69, 89–106

Aim

To examine the effects of work stressors on the individual and the impact on their marital partner.

Method

A questionnaire.

Participants

Participants were recruited via publicity through the University of Herefordshire Alumni Association Newsletter. They were required to be married or cohabiting and both working full time. A total of 27 couples responded, of whom 21 completed the preliminary questionnaire and 20 went on to complete the three weeks of daily questionnaires.

Procedure

Participants completed a preliminary questionnaire plus a daily diary questionnaire every evening for three weeks. The preliminary questionnaire included items relating to:
1) background information
2) measures of work perception e.g. work demands, work relationships, feelings about job
3) anxiety and depression
4) perceived carry-over of work problems to home.
Daily diary questionnaires included items relating to:
1) sleep quality
2) work stressors e.g. demands and support
3) domestic stressors
4) cognitive symptoms e.g. headaches, concentration or memory problems
5) evening mood
6) communication i.e. work-related discussions at home
7) daily incidents.
The questionnaires were designed to investigate the following issues:
1) daily fluctuations in patterns of mood and sleep for individuals throughout the week
2) within-subject relationships between each individual's work stressors and their daily mood symptoms, taking into account the previous day's mood and symptoms
3) relationships between partners' moods on a day-to-day basis and the extent to which these fluctuations can be predicted from the work and domestic stressors of either partner, taking into account the previous day's mood and symptoms
4) the role played by verbal communication (or the lack of it) about work
5) the factors which predict mood in couples with congruent moods.

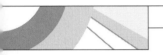

There was no clear evidence of worse mood ratings for Monday than for other days, but weekends had significantly better mood ratings. Sleep was significantly worse on Sunday evenings. Men's evening mood was primarily determined by work stressors, whereas women's evening mood was determined by domestic stress. There was evidence that work stressors spill over into the home. Daily events accounted for more of the variation in female moods and symptoms than in male moods, particularly events relating to interpersonal relationships. The study did not show any direct relationship between individual work stressors and partners' moods. Even for those days rated as particularly stressful, stressors were related to an individual's own evening mood, but not directly related to their partner's mood.

Evaluating research into quality of working life

Questionnaires

All three studies described in this section involve the use of questionnaires. The Swanson *et al.* study used questionnaires to gather data about occupational stress and family life in doctors, Wright and Cropanzano used various questionnaires to assess the impact of emotional exhaustion on job performance and Jones and Fletcher asked participants to complete questionnaires relating to work stress and its impact on marital partners. As a research tool, questionnaires have both advantages and disadvantages. The advantages include the fact that they are easy to administer, generally quick to complete and large sets of data can be gathered in a relatively short space of time. The data from questionnaires are often quantitative and are easily analysed and compared. The main disadvantage of questionnaires is the potential for bias. Participants are likely to be aware that they are participating in some form of research and that the results of the questionnaire will be assessed or evaluated in some way. Hence they are likely to respond to demand characteristics where they answer in the way they think is expected of them by the experimenter or they may show a social desirability bias where they answer so as to show themselves in the best light rather than answering honestly.

Longitudinal research

The Wright and Cropanzano study was carried out over a period of one year and the Jones and Fletcher study was conducted for three weeks. Both studies could be considered longitudinal as they look at ways in which behaviour and experience change over the course of time. This method has advantages over cross-sectional or snapshot studies, where researchers study participants at a particular point in time. Wright and Cropanzano were able to measure changes in emotional exhaustion, job satisfaction and performance during the year. They were also able to monitor voluntary turnover during that period. In the Jones and Fletcher study daily questionnaires were completed over a three-week period, which will have generated far more data than a snapshot study, as well as providing a far more realistic picture of work stress and its impact on marital relationships. The disadvantages of longitudinal research are that they are time-consuming and expensive and may suffer from subject attrition, where participants withdraw from the study.

Sampling

The sample in the study by Jones and Fletcher were volunteers recruited through advertisements. This could be regarded as a biased sample as the majority of the population is unlikely to volunteer to participate in research, and those who do may be atypical of the target population in some way. The advertisement was placed in the University of Herefordshire Alumni Association Newsletter, a further source of bias, as only certain groups of people would have access to such a publication. The sample is also relatively small, comprising just 27 couples.

In contrast, the sample in the Swanson *et al.* study is very large, including 986 doctors from Scottish Health Boards. A sample of this size is far more likely to be representative. However, the results can only be generalized to similar health professionals as other professions would involve different work commitments and occupational stress. It is also questionable whether the results can be generalized to other Health Boards, as Scottish Health Boards may differ from those in other parts of the country.

In the Wright and Cropanzano study the sample comprised graduate social welfare workers. There would be limits to the extent to which these results could be generalized to other occupations or to people with lower levels of educational attainment. There is also a gender bias in this sample, with only 31 per cent being female.

Applications/usefulness

The value of these studies is that they highlight the negative effects of occupational stress. The studies show that work stress can affect job performance and job satisfaction, as well as spilling over into home life and relationships. The Jones and Fletcher study suggests that there are gender differences, with domestic stress having more of an impact on females. However, the Swanson *et al.* study found that increasing domestic role demands were related to stress for both male and female doctors. The study by Wright and Cropanzano suggests that emotional exhaustion is likely to lead to voluntary withdrawal from the organization. Research of this nature should be of use to employers concerned for the welfare of their staff and for the success of their organization. Reducing stress on employees is likely to make them happier, more effective and more satisfied and may also reduce the likelihood of them leaving the organization.

STUDY 80
Fried, Y., Melamed, S., Ben-David, H. A., 2002, 'The joint effects of noise, job complexity, and gender on employee sickness absence: an exploratory study across 21 organizations – the CORDIS study', *Journal of Occupational and Organizational Psychology*, 75, 131–44

Aim

This study is part of the CORDIS study (Cardiovascular Occupational Risk Factors Determination in Israel). In this article the authors examine the joint effects of noise, job complexity and gender on sickness absence.

Method

A correlational study using a range of measures.

Participants

880 white-collar employees of 21 different manufacturing organizations in Israel – six textile, five heavy metal, two light metal, three plywood/Formica, two electronics, two food products and one printing organization.

The sample comprised 396 males and 484 females, with an average age of 38 years. They worked as computer programmers, engineers, lab technicians, secretaries, accounts clerks and chemists.

Procedure

Noise levels in each workplace were measured using a sound meter. Noise levels were sampled twice a day for 30 minutes, with measurements taken in both summer and winter. Results were recorded in decibels and a mean was calculated.

Job complexity was measured by expert raters, who observed workers in their jobs for a whole day. Job complexity was measured by four scales: decisions, skill level, independence and sophistication, and each was rated on a 4-point scale (1 = simple, 4 = complex). A further rating of job variety (1 = no diversity, 4 = lots of diverse tasks) was also recorded. The authors report that job complexity and variety correlated positively at 0.87 (on the standard scale of 0–1) and inter-rater reliability across three observers was very high (0.91).

Sickness absence was monitored for two years (1985–7). The number of absences and the total number of days was recorded.

The authors also note in their procedure that there were no gender differences in job complexity, although women were exposed to slightly higher levels of noise in their jobs (64.9 decibels versus 61.5 decibels).

Results

Both noise and gender are positively correlated with sickness absence. In other words, the higher the levels of noise employees were exposed to, the more absences they had and overall women had more absences than men. However, job complexity was negatively correlated with absences, suggesting that employees with more complex jobs were less likely to be absent due to sickness.

A more detailed analysis of the results showed that it was women in high complexity jobs who showed the strongest association between noise and absence.

For males and females in low complexity jobs this association was not evident.

The authors conclude that the results offer support for the notion that noise and job complexity are detrimental to employee health, especially for women and they speculate that men may pay an even higher price by failing to take care of their health at earlier stages. They suggest that exposure to high levels of noise may produce higher rates of sickness absence for males if the data were to be collected over a longer period of time.

STUDY 81
Bohle, P., Tilley, A., 1998, 'Early experiences of shift work: influences on attitudes', *Journal of Occupational and Organizational Psychology*, 71, 61–79

Aim

The aim of this study was to examine attitudes towards irregular, rapid-rotation shift work and to identify the factors that predicted dissatisfaction with shift work.

Method

A longitudinal study, using a variety of personality tests and attitude scales at three points during the 15 months: on starting shift work, after six months and after 15 months.

Participants

130 female trainee nurses were studied during their first 15 months of shift work. They were aged between 17 and 40 years, with a mean age of just under 20 years. They were all working in hospitals in Australia.

48 of the trainees worked a two-shift roster, involving day shifts (starting between 06.45 and 09.00) and afternoon shifts (starting between 13.00 and 14.45). They worked four days or fewer on each shift and sometimes changed shift day to day. The other 82 trainees had started on a two-shift roster, as above, but had been transferred to a three-shift roster after six months. This involved night shifts starting between 22.00 and 23.00 and trainees worked two to five night shifts at a time. All shifts were 8.5 hours in length and overtime was rare.

Procedure

All trainees completed a range of personality tests at the start of the study. These included the Eysenck Personality Inventory (measuring introversion–extroversion and neuroticism), a Circadian Type Questionnaire, a Social Support Scale and a General Health Questionnaire. No differences were found between the two-shift and the three-shift group on these measures.

Trainees were also asked to respond to a number of statements measuring perceived conflict between shift work and non-work activities. These included the following statements, which had to be rated on a scale of 1–5 (1 = completely false, 5 = completely true): 'Shift work allows me sufficient time for social activities', 'Shift work does not allow me enough time at home', 'Shift work prevents me from participating in sport and leisure activities', 'My family and friends complain because shift work does not allow me to spend enough time with them' and 'Shift-work leaves me with enough free time'. Trainees were also asked to respond to a number of statements measuring attitudes to shift work. The key question was: 'On the whole, how do you feel about working shifts?' This had to be answered on a 5-point scale (1 = I like it very much, 5 = I dislike it very much). The same question was also asked for each of the three shifts (morning, afternoon and evening).

Results

Not surprisingly, night shifts were rated the most negatively and were associated with increased fatigue, sleep disturbances and gastrointestinal complaints. However, positive aspects to working nights were also identified by the trainee nurses and this included the findings that night shifts tended to be more peaceful and allow for more independent working.

A number of variables predicted dissatisfaction with shift working and the most important of these were conflicts between work and non-work activities, the level of social support available to the individual and the number of negative physical effects experienced. However, in this study dissatisfaction scores were relatively low and changed little throughout the 15 months of the study. There were no differences found between the attitudes of the two-shift group and those of the three-shift group. It is possible that these findings are due to the particular sample being studied here (this is discussed below).

STUDY 82
Oldham, G. R., Fried, Y., 1987, 'Employee reactions to workplace characteristics', *Journal of Applied Psychology*, 72, 1, 75–80

| Aim | To investigate the effect of four workplace characteristics on three measures of employee reactions. The four workplace characteristics were: social density, room darkness, number of enclosures and interpersonal distance. The three employee reactions were: staff turnover, satisfaction with job and withdrawal from office during break periods. |

Method

A combination of observational and self-report measures.

Participants

109 clerical employees from different offices in a large university in the USA. 101 of the employees were female and only eight were male.

Procedure

The workplace characteristics were measured as follows:
1) social density – this was a simple measure of the number of employees that worked in each office
2) darkness – this was rated by the researchers on a 3-point scale, from light to dark
3) number of enclosures – this was measured by counting the number of walls and enclosures that surrounded each employee's desk
4) interpersonal distance – this was a measure of the distance between the employee's desk and the nearest co-worker's desk.

Note that two of these measures (social density and darkness) are measures of the workplace as a whole and, as such, are the same for each employee in that office. The other measures are individual measures and would vary for each employee within an office.

The employee reactions were measured as follows:
1) staff turnover – approximately 24 months after data on the workplace characteristics were collected, the number of staff leaving each office was obtained from personnel records
2) satisfaction with job – a questionnaire based on the Job Diagnostic Survey was administered to each participant (this gave a measure of how satisfied each participant was with their job)
3) withdrawal from office during break periods – participants were asked where they usually spent their coffee breaks (i.e. in the office or elsewhere).

Results

The results suggest that workplace characteristics have an effect on the behaviour and attitudes of employees. When offices were dark, there were fewer enclosures around a desk, employees were seated very close to each other and there were lots of workers in the office, participants were more likely to rate themselves as dissatisfied with their work and more likely to withdraw from the office during break periods. Improvements on any one of the four workplace characteristics had significant positive effects on these reactions. Staff turnover was also higher when the office characteristics were more negative.

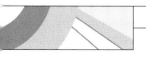

Evaluating research into organizational work conditions

Validity of rating scales

The study by Fried *et al.* rated job complexity at the 'job' level rather than at an individual level. This gives a general indication of how complex each job was but does not tell us precisely how complex each worker found their job. This may reduce the validity of this measure. If individuals were asked to rate how complex they found their jobs, this might generate very different results. It could be argued that the validity would be higher as individuals are actually giving their own opinions, but factors such as demand characteristics may lower the validity as individuals may feel unwilling to state that they find their job overly complex (or too easy) – perhaps individuals could be rated rather than jobs. In a similar way, Oldham and Fried rated the workplace characteristics by observation. Once again, asking participants for their subjective ratings of these characteristics may have generated different results. In contrast, the research by Bohle and Tilley asked trainee nurses to rate their satisfaction with their jobs. This may be a valid measure, but again there are factors which may mean that these participants did not give accurate answers. As trainees, they may have felt uncomfortable with stating that they were dissatisfied in their work and may have felt that such comments could have negative repercussions. Finally, nursing may be very different from other occupations and this may reduce the generalizability of the findings.

Generalization

The study by Fried *et al.* was conducted in Israel, the study by Bohle and Tilley in Australia and the study by Oldham and Fried in the USA. It may be that cultural differences prevent this type of research from being generalized to other cultures. This would be supported by the research in the 'Interpersonal communication' section of this chapter, which suggests that different countries have very different expectations of working conditions. Further, the research described in this section was conducted on very different occupations. Bohle and Tilley have looked at attitudes to shift work among student nurses and there are a number of reasons why this sample may respond differently to other samples. First, anyone considering nursing as a profession will be well aware that shift work is likely to be part of their job, at least in the initial stages, and this may explain why this sample is less dissatisfied with shift work than might be predicted. Further, they have not been working shifts for very long and workers who have worked shifts for several years may have very different attitudes to their work. Fried *et al.* describe their sample as white-collar workers and it may be that workers in other kinds of occupations respond differently to variables such as noise and job complexity. Finally, Oldham and Fried studied clerical workers in universities and it may be that their results would generalize to other similar institutions, but again, it should not be concluded that all workers will respond in the same way to these workplace characteristics. If you sit at the same desk all the time, you may be affected differently by these characteristics than if you had a job which involved a lot of moving about or being in different places all the time. Finally, there are significant gender issues in this kind of research.

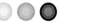

Gender

Females respond differently to noise and other environmental conditions than males. This is shown in a number of studies outlined in the Environment chapter of this book. Specifically, it would seem that women are more negatively affected by adverse environmental factors. The research by Fried *et al.* confirms this finding. However, the research by Oldham and Fried has concentrated on female clerical workers. It may be that the women they studied respond more negatively to social density, room darkness, lack of enclosures and interpersonal distance than men might.

There may also be cultural differences to consider here. The role of women in Israel may be different to the role of women in Australia and the USA. This might explain some of the results found here. Alternatively, there may be common factors between cultures, such as childcare pressures, which mean that women take more time off work than men or find the conflicts between work and domestic responsibilities more difficult to deal with. It is interesting in the light of this to consider the relatively low rates of dissatisfaction reported by Bohle and Tilley in their research with student nurses. While we might expect women to suffer more from work/non-work conflicts than men, this was not shown in this research. It is probable that the very young age of the trainees explains this. It would be interesting to compare these results with a study looking at shift work in groups of women with children and other domestic responsibilities.

Usefulness

There are many useful applications of these research studies. The study by Fried *et al.* suggests that ways need to be found to ensure that workplaces are quieter. This would appear to have particular benefits for women and those with complex jobs. Obviously this is not going to be possible in many workplaces due the nature of the work going on, but recognizing the effects of constant exposure to noise is important and it may be possible to find coping strategies to help people deal with noise.

Oldham and Fried's study has several useful applications. In general terms, this research would suggest that large, bright offices, with enclosures between desks would produce more satisfied staff. However, given the points made above, this may only be the case for female workers with primarily desk-based jobs. Bohle and Tilley's research has limited applications outside the nursing profession. However, they do identify a number of factors which appear to affect levels of satisfaction with shift work and raising awareness of these factors among new trainees may be beneficial.

See also...	

Studies 5, 6, 7, 35, 52, 53, 54, 85, 117, 125, 126 and 128.

Section 4
ENVIRONMENT

ENVIRONMENT
Environmental stress – noise

STUDY 83
Abey-Wickrama, I., A'Brook, M. F., Gattoni, F. E. G., Herridge, C. F., 1969, 'Mental hospital admissions and aircraft noise', *The Lancet*, 13, 1275–7

Aim

To investigate the relationship between aircraft noise and mental health problems. The researchers predicted that there would be higher rates of admissions to mental hospitals from a population living within the maximum noise area – defined as sound levels above 100 PNdB (perceived noise in decibels) – around Heathrow Airport.

Method

A natural experiment. The independent variable was the area in which people live.

Participants

124,000 people over the age of 14 living in or outside the maximum noise area. The two populations were similar in terms of age, sex, marital status and population density. Slight differences were found in terms of socio-economic status and migration, but these differences would predict, if anything, greater levels of mental health problems in the population outside the maximum noise area.

Procedure

A retrospective study looking at mental hospital admissions in the area over the previous two years and comparing the population living within the maximum noise area with the population living outside the maximum noise area.

Results

The results showed a significant difference between mental hospital admissions in the two areas. People living within the maximum noise area were significantly more likely to be admitted to mental hospitals. This effect was particularly strong for 'older women not living with husband' and for those with a history of neurosis. The authors concluded that while they have not demonstrated a causal link between aircraft noise and mental health admissions, they have shown that aircraft noise is likely to be a factor explaining increased hospital admissions.

STUDY 84
McElrea, H., Standing, L., 1992, 'Fast music causes fast drinking', *Perceptual and Motor Skills*, 75, 362

| Aim | To test the hypothesis that the tempo (speed) of music will affect drinking time. |

Aim   To test the hypothesis that the tempo (speed) of music will affect drinking time.

Method   A laboratory experiment with independent measures.

Participants   140 female undergraduates.

Procedure   Participants were randomly assigned to one of two conditions (fast or slow music condition). The music was a recording of the same medley of songs (details not given in the report) played either quickly or slowly on a piano (132 or 54 beats on a metronome). The music was played at 'quiet background levels'. Subjects were tested in groups of five and were simply asked to drink a can of soda and to rate its flavour (mild deception). Participants were observed and the time taken to drink the can was recorded.

Results   There was a significant difference between the drinking times of each condition. Participants drank their soda slower when the music was slow and drank their soda faster when the music was fast. The researchers therefore concluded that the tempo of music significantly affects drinking time.

STUDY 85

Evans, G. W., Johnson, D., 2000, 'Stress and open-office noise', *Journal of Applied Psychology*, 85, 5, 779–83

| Aim | To investigate the effects of simulated open-office noise on a number of physiological and behavioural variables. |

Aim

To investigate the effects of simulated open-office noise on a number of physiological and behavioural variables.

Method

A laboratory experiment with repeated measures (control condition compared to experimental condition).

Participants

40 female clerical workers with a mean age of 36.5 years. They were recruited through advertisements in local newspapers and were paid $150 for their participation. The study was described to them as a research project on computer workstation equipment.

Procedure

Participants were tested at the Cornell Human Factors Laboratory in simulated office environments. Each participant took part in two experimental sessions, a three-hour clerical work session and a three-hour resting baseline session (conducted one to three days later). In the first session, participants worked at a variety of clerical tasks under either quiet or simulated noise conditions. The noise consisted of conversation fragments, ringing phones, typing noises and drawers being opened and closed. These noises had been recorded and were played over loudspeakers. Participants were also asked to drink a glass of water every 25 minutes during both three-hour sessions, so that urine could be collected for physiological testing.

A number of dependent measures were used in this study. These included levels of epinephrine (high levels = stress), norepinephrine (high levels = physical exertion) and cortisol (high levels = psychological distress), number of adjustments made to workstation (moving chair, monitor, keyboard etc.), number of words typed per minute and number of errors made. Participants also completed self-reports on perceived noise and feelings of stress. Finally, a set of puzzles (including some that were unsolvable) were used to test levels of motivation.

Results

Participants in the open-office noise condition perceived the environment as significantly noisier than participants in the quiet environment. Typing speed and number of mistakes were not affected by noise. There was no significant difference in the self-reports of perceived stress, but there were significantly higher levels of epinephrine in the noisy condition. Participants showed higher levels of stress in the motivation task, with those in the noisy condition making significantly fewer attempts to solve the puzzles. Finally, participants made fewer movements in the noisy condition. The researchers concluded that simulated office noise does have a negative effect on participants.

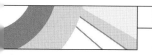

Evaluating research into environmental stress – noise

Research methods/level of control over variables

These three studies use a range of different research methods and therefore have differing levels of control over variables. The study by Abey-Wickrama et al. is a 'natural experiment' as there is no attempt to control or manipulate variables and the researchers are taking advantage of a 'naturally occurring variable' – whether people are living inside or outside a maximum noise area around Heathrow Airport. This means that the researchers do not have the ability to control for any other variables that might influence mental hospital admissions, although they do recognize this problem and suggest which other variables might bear further examination. In contrast, in the studies by McElrea and Standing and Evans and Johnson there are much higher levels of control as these studies are conducted in laboratory situations. In particular, the study by Evans and Johnson demonstrated high levels of control over all variables: the same background noise was played to each participant and each participant drank the same amount of water at regular intervals and was tested using the same tasks.

The ability to isolate and control variables is a strength of laboratory research as it reduces the possibility of confounding variables and strengthens the likelihood that the independent variable is having an effect on the dependent variable. This further reduces the likelihood that other variables may be responsible for the results. As we mentioned above, this may be particularly true of the research by Abey-Wickrama et al. They identify the mediating effect of gender, living alone and a history of neurosis on likelihood of being admitted to hospital. Given the nature of this kind of research, this 'other variable effect' is to be expected and it would obviously be unethical to conduct the kind of experimental research that would offer 'cause and effect' conclusions here. In contrast, the laboratory study by Evans and Johnson does manage to isolate the variable office noise by recording this and playing it through loudspeakers. However, office noise is never experienced like this and would usually also involve the presence of other people, the invasion of personal space and so on. In this situation the researchers have achieved high levels of control, but this may have been at the expense of ecological validity.

Ecological validity

We have said that high levels of control in laboratory situations may be associated with low levels of ecological validity and the reverse is true of research conducted in more natural settings. This means that the research by Abey-Wickrama et al. has high levels of ecological validity as it was conducted in a real situation measuring real variables (admissions to mental hospitals). In contrast, the study by McElrea and Standing is artificial and bears little resemblance to real life. Although there are undoubtedly real-life applications of this study, it should be remembered that this study asked participants to sit in a room on their own and drink a can of soda. Most often people would have a coffee or a drink with others in a social situation and this would be just one of a number of other variables that might influence the relationship between tempo of music and drinking speed. While it may be tempting to apply these results to speed of drinking alcohol in nightclubs, for example, you should remember that this is not what the researchers tested. The ecological validity of the study by Evans and Johnson is more difficult to assess. In some respects it has very high ecological validity. The researchers are testing office workers in office environments and this can obviously be seen as having high ecological validity. However, the participants were not in their normal office environments, they knew they were being observed and the office noise was being played on speakers; these factors, together with the use of regular physiological tests, may have increased the artificiality of the situation and hence their behaviour.

Gender

There is an interesting gender issue arising from these studies. Both the laboratory studies (McElrea and Standing, Evans and Johnson) use only female participants. It could be argued that this significantly reduces the generalizability of this research to males. It is possible that males are less (or more, or differently) affected by music or noise and further research would be necessary to answer this question. Interestingly, the study by Abey-Wickrama *et al.* contributes to this issue as they identify the combination of variables – being female and living alone – as a major mediating effect. In other words, they are saying that being female and living alone has an influence on the way in which you are affected by noise.

As you read the rest of the research described in this chapter you will find that this gender issue occurs repeatedly. It would appear that females are more affected by a number of environmental variables and perhaps this will prove to be a future focus for researchers working in this field.

Usefulness

All three studies described in this section have useful applications. Clearly the research by Abey-Wickrama *et al.* would suggest either that airports should be sited at a considerable distance from housing or that there is a need for practical help for people who live within maximum noise areas. This could be in the form of increased double glazing and other sound-insulating techniques or in the form of coping strategies for individuals. At the very least this research suggests that it might be possible to identify those who are at highest risk of mental health problems and develop some form of intervention. The study by McElrea and Standing could be applied to cafes or restaurants that wished people to eat or drink faster (either so they buy more or so they can have a faster turnover of customers). This research would suggest that playing fast music in this environment would have this effect (although see the reservations above about people alone versus in groups). It could even be suggested by policy makers who want to encourage people to drink less, although the application might prove difficult. Finally, despite the comments made about the ecological validity of the research by Evans and Johnson, it is clear that this research would suggest that work is less effective and workers more stressed in large open-plan offices and this may have several useful applications for those involved in designing office accommodation.

ENVIRONMENT
Climate and weather

STUDY 86
Michael, R. P., Zumpe, D., 1986, 'An annual rhythm in the battering of women', *American Journal of Psychiatry*, 143, 5

| Aim | To investigate the hypothesis that violence by men against women increases in the summer. |

Aim

To investigate the hypothesis that violence by men against women increases in the summer.

Method

A correlational study (investigating the relationship between temperature and rates of violence).

Participants

Analysis of 27,000 reports of women abused by live-in male partners. Reports were provided by 23 shelter organizations in five areas of the USA (Atlanta, Texas, Oregon, Wyoming and California) and covered a period of approximately two years.

Procedure

Mean monthly temperatures for the relevant years were obtained from the National Climatic Center. These were compared to the reports of violence to see if any patterns emerged.

Results

In all the areas studied, there was a relationship between temperature and number of reports of violent activity. Violence increased very significantly during the summer months, with peaks occurring at approximately 80 degrees Fahrenheit. The authors conclude that this may be due to a direct effect of temperature on human irritability or possibly to a neuro-endocrine mechanism, involving neural pathways, which is affected by seasonal factors. Interestingly, the authors also point out that other research has shown strong seasonal patterns of violence against children with peaks at very different times of the year.

STUDY 87

Carskadon, M. A., Acebo, C., 1993, 'Parental reports of seasonal mood and behavior changes in children', *Journal of American Academy of Child and Adolescent Psychiatry*, 32, 2, 264–9

Aim

This study aimed to investigate seasonal behavioural changes in children.

Method

A survey.

Participants

The parents of 892 girls and 788 boys aged 9–11 years were asked to participate. All the children lived in the USA.

Procedure

Parents were asked to complete a checklist of seasonal behavioural symptoms. These were as follows: negative sleeping patterns, negative eating patterns, irritability, lack of energy, withdrawal and sadness. Parents were asked to indicate how frequent these behavioural symptoms were in each season.

Results

At least one negative symptom was reported in winter for 49 per cent of children. This compared to only 9 per cent in autumn and 11 per cent in spring.

More girls were reported to be tired in winter, but otherwise there were no differences between the sexes. Age effects were found for girls with increased prevalence of tiredness and withdrawal in older girls in winter. Finally, the children living in the northern states of the USA were reported to show more winter symptoms than those living in the southern states. The researchers concluded that seasonality effects are common in children and that these symptoms need more careful research. They also point to the possible beneficial effects of light therapy.

STUDY 88

Kasper, S. *et al.*, 1989, 'Epidemiological findings of seasonal changes in mood and behaviour. A telephone survey of Montgomery County, Maryland', *Archives of General Psychiatry*, 46, 9, 823–33

Aim	To assess the prevalence of seasonal changes in mood and behaviour.
Method	A survey.
Participants	Randomly selected households in Montgomery County, MD, USA. The method of random sampling was random telephone digit dialling.
Procedure	Participants who agreed to participate were questioned over the phone using the Seasonal Pattern Assessment Questionnaire, which examines a range of behavioural and mood symptoms that have been associated with seasonality effects.
Results	Over 92 per cent of those questioned noticed seasonality effects on their mood and behaviour. 27 per cent of the sample described seasonal changes as a problem for them and 5–10 per cent exhibited symptoms equivalent to patients diagnosed as suffering from Seasonal Affective Disorder (SAD). Finally, more women exhibited symptoms than men. The researchers conclude that SAD may be just the extreme end of the 'spectrum of seasonality' that affects the vast majority of the population. They suggest that further research into seasonality effects may provide useful insights into mental health more generally.

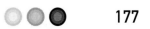

> **STUDY 89**
> Michalak, E. *et al.*, 2003, 'Seasonality, negative life events and social support in a community sample', *British Journal of Psychiatry*, 182, 434–8

Aim

To investigate the association between psychosocial variables and reported seasonal patterns of mood disorder and Seasonal Affective Disorder (SAD).

Method

A correlation using questionnaires/interviews to measure variables.

Participants

1250 people aged 18–64 years, drawn randomly from North Wales Health Authority GP database.

Procedure

All participants were sent a postal questionnaire. This was a sub-scale of the SPAQ (seasonal patterns assessment questionnaire), which gives a global seasonality score (GSS). This score indicates the amount of change that an individual experiences in sleep patterns, mood, weight, appetite, energy and social activity. The scale's range is 0–24, with scores of 11 and above indicating a moderate problem. Participants were also asked to complete a checklist of recent (last six months) negative life experiences and a questionnaire measuring levels of social support and answer a series of basic demographic questions.

All participants scoring 11+ on the SPAQ (66 participants) were asked to take part in a further diagnostic interview. 55 of these participants agreed and 25 were diagnosed as suffering from SAD.

Results

Several variables correlated strongly with SPAQ scores. These were as follows:
1) having experienced high numbers of negative life events in the last six months
2) having a poorer social support network
3) being female
4) being born outside the area.
Overall, despite a small sample and questions over the validity of the scales, these results offer strong support for the role of psychosocial factors in seasonality effects.

Evaluating research into climate and weather

Types of data collection
The research described in this section has used two forms of data collection. The study by Michael and Zumpe has used statistical information collected from shelter organizations and the other three studies have used questionnaire/survey methods. The use of statistical data is common in environmental research as it allows researchers to study genuine effects rather than laboratory-based effects, which may lack ecological validity. However, you could consider if the data collected here is an accurate measure of violence and threats of violence. Not all violent acts are reported to shelter organizations and it is probable that many violent acts or threats of violence go unreported. However, the researchers are aware of this problem and are using the data as a way of showing how these figures change with the temperature

rather than suggesting that they are an accurate measure of violent activity. Unless people are more likely to report violence and threats of violence in certain temperatures (which seems unlikely), they have demonstrated that a correlation exists. Also it would not be possible to conduct experimental research on this for very obvious practical and ethical reasons. Researchers have no control over the temperature and to conduct a piece of research which set out to manipulate violent behaviour would be highly unethical. Kasper *et al.* and Michalak *et al.* asked people to report their own symptoms via either a telephone or postal questionnaire. This has some disadvantages as people may not give accurate information, it is not possible to explore answers in more detail and, in the case of the postal questionnaire, the person you wanted to complete the questionnaire may not be the one who actually does so. However, a questionnaire may be less intrusive and more confidential than asking people to answer these questions face to face. Finally, Carskadon and Acebo asked parents to report on observed seasonality effects; while this is an appropriate way to find about children's behaviour, it may be less accurate than asking children themselves and parents may give false information for a number of reasons.

Correlational research/control over variables

Research into the relationship between weather and behaviour is correlational. That is, the results demonstrate a relationship between the variables and do not demonstrate that one variable causes a change in the other. This is not to say that there is no cause-and-effect relationship, but that without conducting experimental research (involving manipulation and control of variables) it is not possible to draw these conclusions. The research by Michael and Zumpe shows this relationship but does not prove that a rise in temperature actually causes a rise in violent activity. There may be a third variable explanation, such as rise in temperature changing people's social activity, which in turn affects violent behaviour, or there may be other variables, such as seasonal stresses to do with employment rates or pollution, which have not been considered. The research by Kasper *et al.* and by Carskadon and Acebo only asked about seasonality effects rather than other seasonal changes in people's lives. Once again, there may be other variables which contribute to the seasonality effects they found. The research by Michalak *et al.* highlights some of these variables. They set out to examine how other variables (negative life events and levels of social support) influenced seasonality effects. They found that a number of factors interact. Their findings mirror those of Abey-Wickrama *et al.* (see study 83, this chapter) in that negative life events, lack of social support and gender contributed to the effects of seasonality. These comments do not detract from the findings reported in this section, but do demonstrate that environmental factors are unlikely to work in isolation, showing complex interactions between environment and psychosocial variables. Finally, it demonstrates the difficulty of isolating variables to study in environmental psychology.

Participants/generalization

The samples used in these studies are worth considering in some detail. Michael and Zumpe collected an enormous 27,000 reports of violence against women in various parts of the USA. While this is clearly a very large sample, it is self-selected in the sense that it is only women who have reported violence and the data may not be an accurate reflection of violence against women in general. Further it is US research and the same seasonality effects may not be found in countries with different climates or different cultures. Michalak *et al.* concentrated their research on one part of the United Kingdom (North Wales), which is predominantly rural. It may be that different results would be found in large inner-city areas or among a different sample. Carskadon and Acebo's research focused on children aged 9–11 years and it may be that age is an important variable when considering these effects.

Usefulness

The research described in this section may have a number of useful applications: it may be worth police departments having more personnel working when the temperature hits the critical values (this does happen in a number of US cities) or it may suggest avenues for further research. As Michael and Zumpe conclude, there may be neurological mechanisms underpinning this effect and further research may provide useful findings. Discovering the huge numbers of people that are affected by seasonal affective disorder (SAD) may encourage the medical profession to take these effects more seriously or may generate research into treatments for SAD. Finally, demonstrating that children are also very influenced by seasonality effects may have useful applications for teachers and those working with children. Identifying times when children's concentration may be impaired or the levels of irritability may be higher could be very useful indeed.

STUDY 90

Nagaraja, H. S., Jeganathan, P. S., 2003, 'Effect of acute and chronic conditions of overcrowding on free choice ethanol intake in rats', *Indian Journal of Physiological Pharmacology*, 47, 3, 325–31

| Aim | To examine the effects of overcrowding on ethanol (alcohol) intake in rats. |

| Method | A laboratory experiment with independent measures and two conditions. |

| Participants | Groups of male albino rats. |

| Procedure | This was a laboratory experiment with independent measures and two conditions:

1) acute stressed group – these rats were kept in overcrowded conditions for a period of six hours per day for seven days
2) chronic stressed group – these rats were kept in continuous overcrowded conditions for seven days.

The rats in both conditions had access to ethanol as well as other liquids and the intake for each group was measured. |

| Results | The rats in the chronic stressed group showed a significant increase in both ethanol intake and ethanol preference (over other liquids) compared to the acute stressed group. The researchers conclude that short-lasting stressors do not significantly increase ethanol drinking behaviour, but that longer-term stressors do cause a significant increase in ethanol drinking behaviour. |

STUDY 91
Schwab, J. J., Nadeau, S. E., Warheit, G. J., 1979, 'Crowding and mental health', *Pavlovian Journal of Biological Science*, 14, 4, 226–33

Aim

To investigate the mental health needs of adults living in Florida, USA.

Method

Survey/questionnaires.

Participants

1645 adults aged 17–92 years, including representative quotas of gender, race, income level and age.

Procedure

All respondents completed a Depression Inventory and the Health Opinion Survey. On both of these scales high scores are associated with higher levels of problems. Data were also collected on crowding levels in the home.

Results

Approximately 8 per cent of the sample was considered to be living in overcrowded conditions. There was a strong association between depression and health scores and overcrowding. This association was particularly strong when other factors were also present, and these included being female, being of childbearing age, being black and being in the low to intermediate income range.

STUDY 92
Evans, G., Lepore, S., 1993, 'Household crowding and social support: a quasi-experimental analysis', *Journal of Personality and Social Psychology*, 65, 2, 308–16

Aim

To examine the effects of high-density living on perceived levels of social support.

Method

An experiment.

Participants

72 college students living in off-campus apartments (39 women, 33 men). They were divided into two groups: high density (typically shared rooms, crowded apartments) and low density (one or more rooms to a person). All the students had been living in this accommodation for approximately eight months and were told that the aim of the research was to evaluate the quality of social relationships in off-campus housing.

Procedure

The authors provide an extremely detailed account of the procedure; briefly, it consisted of the following. Participants were tested in a classroom environment. One participant was tested at a time with a confederate whom the participant believed to be another participant. The confederate was blind to the housing condition of the participant. Both participant and confederate were given five minutes to write an essay on political changes in the Soviet Union. They were then allowed to interact (confederate trained to be friendly and responsive). Blood pressure was then measured. The researchers gave feedback on the essays. The confederate was given a mark of 90 (A-) and the participant a mark of 79 (C+). Half the participants were then given social support (positive reassuring comments) from the confederate. The other half of the participants did not receive this support. The participant was then asked privately to rate the supportiveness of the confederate and the confederate was asked to rate the amount of support-seeking by the participant.

In the second part of the study both participant and confederate wrote an essay on the fall of the Berlin Wall. Blood pressure was monitored after this. This time the participant was given a mark of 92 (A-) and the confederate a mark of 79 (C+). The confederate and participant were then left in the room for three minutes. This was to observe the extent to which the participant would be socially supportive towards the confederate. Finally, the experimenter returned and debriefed the participant.

Note that there are three distinct measures being taken in this study:
1) subject's self-reports of confederate's supportiveness
2) confederate's ratings of behaviour
3) observer's ratings of behaviour.

Results

Those participants living in high-density accommodation were less likely to seek support from the confederate after their feedback and also perceived that less support was offered to them by the confederate. In the second phase of the experiment, when the confederate needed social support, participants from high-density accommodation offered less support to the confederate than the participants from lower-density accommodation. Both confederate ratings and observer ratings agreed in this respect. The authors conclude that high-density living has a negative effect on social interaction and suggest that this is due to withdrawal from social interaction in crowded environments as a coping strategy.

STUDY 93
Rotton, J., 1987, 'Hemmed in and hating it: effects of shape of room on tolerance for crowding', *Perceptual and Motor Skills*, 64, 285–6

| Aim | To examine the hypothesis that individuals are less tolerant of crowding in rooms with curved walls than straight walls. This study was undertaken to evaluate a design that had been proposed for a student housing project. The design included an impressive curved wall around a lagoon. Several members of a student housing committee suggested that curved walls might make people feel 'hemmed in'. The researchers therefore propose that curved walls reduce our tolerance for crowding, regardless of whether the wall was concave or convex. |

Aim

To examine the hypothesis that individuals are less tolerant of crowding in rooms with curved walls than straight walls. This study was undertaken to evaluate a design that had been proposed for a student housing project. The design included an impressive curved wall around a lagoon. Several members of a student housing committee suggested that curved walls might make people feel 'hemmed in'. The researchers therefore propose that curved walls reduce our tolerance for crowding, regardless of whether the wall was concave or convex.

Method

A laboratory experiment.

Participants

32 undergraduates (16 men, 16 women).

Procedure

Three model rooms were created from cardboard. These were on a scale of 12:1 and wall heights were approximately 9 cm.
    Room 1 = square room, 38 x 38 cm
    Room 2 = circular, with a radius of 22.6 cm
    Room 3 = measured 42 cm on three sides, but had one concave wall with a 60 degree arc.
    The task was to place figures 5.7 cm high into the rooms until the addition of one more would make the room crowded. Participants completed each task twice for each room, once assuming that the model figures were friends and once assuming that they were acquaintances. Order of trial was counterbalanced.

Results

Significantly more figures were placed in the room when they represented friends than when they represented acquaintances (mean for friends = 11, mean for acquaintances = 8.9). Participants also put more figures in the square room (mean = 10.9) than the circular room (mean = 8). There was no significant difference between the mean number of figures placed in the circular room and the room with the concave wall, although the difference was 'approaching significance' and the researchers conclude that they have support for the idea that individuals are less tolerant of crowding in rooms with curved walls than straight walls.

Evaluating research into density and crowding

Control over variables
There are a number of issues to consider here. The first is the application of animal research to the explanation of human behaviour. There are a number of reasons why a researcher might choose to use animals as research subjects rather than humans and the major one we will discuss here is the ability to control the environment and confounding variables (we will discuss ethical issues later).

    It is possible to breed rats for research and ensure that you have a sample which have identical environments up until the point of the study. Therefore you have a level of control in the research that would be impossible to achieve in human research. If you conducted this study with humans you would not be able to control people's life experiences, levels of stress and a host of other factors that might contribute to their alcohol intake to a greater extent than the variable of overcrowding. So in this sense, Nagaraja and Jeganathan's research is highly controlled and they can be reasonably safe in concluding that it was the level of crowding that contributed to the level of alcohol intake. In contrast, there is not the same level of control over confounding variables in the research by Evans and Lepore. Although they have clearly defined experimental groups (shared rooms versus single rooms), there are a number of other factors that may influence the levels of social support sought and offered. These might include whether the participants had their own room at home, the size of their families, the level of social support at home and whether they had expressed a preference for single or shared accommodation. This does not detract from the conclusions reached by the researchers, but demonstrates the difficulty of isolating variables in environmental research. Schwab *et al.*'s research confirms this by once again demonstrating a complex interaction between variables.

Ecological validity/application to real life

There are a number of issues related to ecological validity and we will consider the research by Rotton first. In this study participants were asked to place model figures into model rooms. It is questionable whether these models can accurately represent real rooms and real people. Rotton recognizes this and, to judge from his conclusion, seems to regard this research as a kind of pilot study, arguing that the results support the need for further research in real-life settings. The research by Evans and Lepore perhaps has higher ecological validity than the research by Rotton as the task (writing essays and receiving feedback on them) is very similar to the real-life experiences of being a student. However, the participants are aware that this is an experiment and this may mean that the effects of negative/positive feedback are heightened (or reduced). Further, the independent variable (single or shared rooms) is a naturally occurring variable and this may add to the validity of the findings, although which type of room people live in may be due to a number of other factors, as discussed above. Finally, how can we assess the ecological validity of the research by Nagaraja and Jeganathan? Rats do not generally have access to alcohol and it is difficult to know what relevance to real life and, in particular, human life this study might have. It would be difficult even to apply this research to the behaviour of rats in the wild as laboratory rats have always lived in highly artificial and controlled environments.

Ethics

All animal research raises ethical issues. There are different ethical guidelines for researchers working with animals and these stress the importance of suitable living environments, adequate food, water and space and forbid researchers from inflicting stress or pain on them. It could be argued that Nagaraja and Jeganathan's research breaks all these guidelines. There is, of course, the wider debate of whether we have the right to use animals for research purposes and there are a number of valid viewpoints here. Perhaps the critical one concerns the necessity or otherwise of this piece of research. Does it add to our understanding of rat behaviour in any way? Does it have anything to tell us about human behaviour? If your answers to these questions are 'no', you would probably agree that this research should not have been conducted.

The research by Evans and Lepore raises a very different ethical issue. Deception of experimental participants and the causing of distress is considered unethical. Arguably, this research does both of those things. Participants were made to feel that their first essays were inadequate compared to those of the confederates and they did not realize that this was a deception. Although you could argue that the reverse situation in the second half of the study may have made the participant feel better, this does not justify the deception. These are not major ethical issues, but they are worth considering. Finally, on a more positive note, the research by Rotton appears to raise no ethical issues at all.

Usefulness

We will start with the research by Evans and Lepore and by Rotton. Both these studies have clear implications for practitioners. In an ideal world, all students should be housed in single rooms, although there are obvious cost implications here. This may be an important piece of research for student counsellors to be aware of, as they may find that they are seeing more students from high-density housing. They could be trained to offer coping strategies or even help arrange for students to move to a different type of accommodation. You would have to guard against self-fulfilling prophecies operating here, however; if students were informed of the negative consequences of shared accommodation this could create further problems. Rotton's research clearly suggests that curved rooms enhance the feeling of being crowded and this may be related to other research that finds that people feel more crowded in rooms without corners. However, the practical applications of Rotton's research are tempered by the fact that this study had very low ecological validity and further real-world research is required. Finally, Nagaraja and Jeganathan's study does perhaps demonstrate one negative effect of crowding (although see comments above) and the research by Schwab et al. certainly does. There are many practical applications of these findings for planners, mental health practitioners and others, but as always the cost would be a major factor in implementing these suggestions.

ENVIRONMENT
Crowds and collective behaviour

STUDY 94
Mann, L., 1981, 'The baiting crowd in episodes of threatened suicide', *Journal of Personality and Social Psychology*, 41, 4, 703–9

| Aim | This paper examines 21 cases in which crowds were present when a disturbed person threatened to jump off a building, bridge or tower. |

Aim

This paper examines 21 cases in which crowds were present when a disturbed person threatened to jump off a building, bridge or tower.

Method

Content analysis.

Participants

The sample of cases was drawn from newspaper reports of suicides and suicide attempts in New York (15 cases), other large US cities (four cases), Johannesburg (one case) and Rome (one case). All the events took place between 1964 and 1979. 'Baiting' was reported in ten of these cases.

Procedure

The newspaper reports for the 21 cases were analysed and the following details recorded:
1) location of incident (e.g. Empire State Building)
2) position of the victim (e.g. tenth-floor window ledge)
3) date and time of day
4) duration of episode
5) crowd size
6) spectator behaviour during the incident.

Results

Some of the important results include:
1) baiting was more common in large crowds (more than 300 people)
2) baiting was more common when it was darker
3) no baiting occurred when the victim and the crowd were in very close proximity (interestingly, neither did it occur when the victim and the crowd were a great distance apart)
4) baiting was more common the longer the incident went on (baiting was most common in the seven incidents that lasted more than two hours)
5) temperature also contributed to baiting behaviour (eight of the ten baiting incidents happened in the summer whereas only four of the non-baiting incidents took place in the same season).

STUDY 95

Latane, B., Darley, J., 1970, *The Unresponsive Bystander: why doesn't he help?*, New York: Appleton-Century-Crofts

Aim

To investigate the concept of diffusion of responsibility in crowd situations. Specifically, this experiment investigates whether the presence of others would make participants more likely or less likely to seek help in an emergency situation.

Method

A laboratory experiment with three independent conditions.

Participants

Male undergraduate students.

Procedure

Students were asked to complete questionnaires and were shown to a room to do this. They were either in the room alone (Condition 1), with two confederates (Condition 2) or with two other participants (Condition 3). While they completed their questionnaires, the researchers pumped white smoke through an air vent in the room. In Condition 2 the confederates were trained to ignore the emergency. As the room filled with smoke they were to glance at it nonchalantly, shrug and return to their questionnaires. The researchers wanted to see how long it would take participants to leave the room and report the emergency.

Results

Where participants were tested alone, they behaved as you might expect. On average they had left the room within two minutes and 75 per cent of them had left within the researchers' six-minute time limit. However, where participants were tested in groups they behaved very differently. At the end of the six minutes only 10 per cent of the participants tested in Condition 2 (with two confederates) had left the room and, surprisingly, this figure rose to only 15 per cent when all three were genuine participants. Latane and Darley report that by the end of the six minutes the smoke was so thick that the participants could not see the far wall of the room. They stayed at their tables, coughing, rubbing their eyes and fanning the smoke away from their paper so they could see the questions! The researchers conclude that the presence of others has a profound effect on our behaviour and we are much less likely to act independently.

> ### STUDY 96
> Brown, B., 2004, 'CCTV in town centres: three case studies', *Police Research Group: Crime Detection and Prevention Series*, Paper 68, Home Office

| Aim | It has been well documented that in public places where large numbers of people can congregate, antisocial behaviours are likely to occur. This may be due to a number of social psychological influences, including conformity and de-individuation. CCTV should have the effect of reducing de-individuation in crowds – if people know they are being observed, they are less likely to be influenced by crowd membership. This paper summarizes the use and effectiveness of CCTV in three British town centres. |

| Method | The method used here was to analyse data from secondary sources such as crime reports. It could also be seen as a kind of natural experiment comparing behaviour pre- and post-CCTV installation. |

| Procedure | Quantitative data was collected on offending patterns and police resource use. The three towns studied in this research were Birmingham, Newcastle and King's Lynn. |

| Results | The author concludes that CCTV was very effective in all three areas. In particular, he comments that CCTV allows police to manage their resources more effectively and the CCTV recordings can be useful as evidence. In relation to offending patterns, significant reductions were found in all three areas. For example, in Newcastle, burglaries were down by 56 per cent and criminal damage down by 34 per cent. The paper concludes that CCTV has a positive effect in reducing antisocial behaviour, particularly in areas where large quantities of people congregate, such as town centres, and in areas used by large numbers of people but not observed, such as car parks. |

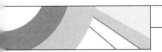

Evaluating research into crowds and collective behaviour

Research methods

Several different research methods were used in the research described in this section. Mann selected newspaper reports of suicides and suicide attempts to analyse. He was able to find ten cases where 'baiting' occurred and a further 11 (from a much larger pool of reports) where it did not. This creates the two groups that are compared. The method is content analysis and there are several strengths and weaknesses associated with this. First, this type of content analysis allows researchers to study events that have happened and cannot be observed or manipulated in any way. However, the results can only be as accurate as the original newspaper article and it is clear that 'baiting' in this type of situation would make a good story and may have been exaggerated by the press. Latane and Darley, in contrast, use an experimental design, including a specially created environment. There are obvious strengths here, including the level of control over variables and the ability to compare directly different experimental conditions. However, this research would also be prone to demand characteristics and low levels of ecological validity.

Ecological validity/application to real life

The research by Brown looks at crime figures and other police data for three towns in England. This has high levels of ecological validity as it examines results from real situations rather than from an artificial laboratory situation. However, it should be remembered that the effects of CCTV reduce over time and this research may need repeating in a few years to check that the results still apply.

This is in contrast to the research by Latane and Darley, which was a highly artificial situation and may have led to people behaving very differently than they might in real life. The use of confederates also reduces ecological validity, although the fact that the people in the group with three naive participants behaved very similarly to the participant in the confederate group might lessen this criticism to some extent.

Ethics/ethical implications

Does this research break ethical guidelines? Clearly the Mann and Brown studies do not harm participants in the same way that the research by Latane and Darley does. The participants in Latane and Darley's research were put into a very stressful situation and may have been very distressed as a result of this. Participants in the confederate condition, in particular, may have been upset by the seeming lack of concern from the confederates. It is clear that such research would require extensive debriefing. Although the other research described here does not raise ethical issues in relation to participants, there are ethical implications of such research. CCTV is controversial and has been criticized for invading privacy. The use of tapes made by CCTV cameras also raises ethical issues.

Usefulness

Taken as a whole, these studies demonstrate the powerful effect that other people can have on our behaviour. This in itself is a useful finding, particularly as the results from the helping behaviour studies are so surprising. Perhaps if the police or others who are involved in large-scale crowd control are made aware of the effects of crowding on behaviour, they would recognize the need to direct people's behaviour more. Mann's results are horrifying and yet it is difficult to imagine how such behaviours could be prevented. Ensuring that crowds of the critical size do not build up when this kind of emergency is taking place is an obvious solution, but it is difficult to imagine how this could be managed effectively. Finally, Brown's study highlights the usefulness of CCTV, but warns that the effects reduce over time and points out that careful consideration needs to be given to placing the cameras.

ENVIRONMENT
Environmental disaster and technological catastrophe

STUDY 97

Havenaar, J. M. *et al.*, 2003, 'Perception of risk and subjective health among victims of the Chernobyl disaster', *Social Science and Medicine*, 56, 569–72

Aim

The nuclear power plant disaster in Chernobyl in 1986 was the largest disaster of its kind. The chain reaction in the nuclear reactor became out of control, causing an explosion and a fireball which blew the steel and concrete lid off the reactor. 30 people died immediately and over 135,000 people living in a 20-mile radius were evacuated. Figures from the Ukraine Radiological Institute suggest that a further 2500 deaths were caused, with the most notable health risk being a rise in the incidence of thyroid cancer, especially in children. There have been several research studies which have shown increased levels of self-reported health problems (other than cancer), psychological distress and use of medical services in the population in the affected area. The researchers claim that the rise in self-reported health problems is not accounted for by clinical health status (in other words, these people do not have more illnesses than a control population) and neither can they be explained by radiation effects. They are proposing that cognitive variables, such as risk perception, sense of control and ratings of credibility of official information, are an important factor in explaining these increases. This research compares these cognitive variables in an affected and an unaffected population.

Method

A natural experiment, as the independent variable (where people live) is a naturally occurring variable. Data were collected through self-report methods.

Participants

Two groups of subjects were compared. The first group comprised 1617 adults from the Gomel region of Belarus, which is considered to be one of the most seriously affected regions in the Chernobyl area. The second group comprised 1427 adults from the Tver region of Russia, an area that is socio-economically comparable to the first, has a nuclear power plant but was not affected by the Chernobyl disaster.

Procedure

All subjects completed a self-report questionnaire, measuring subjective health, psychological distress and contacts with medical services. The questionnaire also contained 5-point Likert items, focusing on:
1) hazard perception
2) sense of control (e.g. In your opinion, to what extent can you personally influence your own and your family's current life situation?)
3) credibility of information (e.g. I trust the information given through the TV, radio and newspapers about the consequences of Chernobyl / I think that the

full extent of the Chernobyl accident is not being told to the public)

4) expectation of recurrence.

| Results |

The people in the Gomel region expressed more concern about the Chernobyl disaster for almost all the cognitive variables. The people in Tver worried more about political and economic issues. This supports the hypothesis that cognitive variables affect levels of self-reported health problems as well as levels of psychological stress and level of medical services use. However, the exact relationship between these variables is unclear. It may be that the stress caused by being in the affected area is enough to explain the rise in these levels. However, the researchers also suggest that exposure to ionizing radiation and the concerns that would inevitably arise from this may stimulate people's awareness of physical sensations and they are more likely to be alarmed by these. Finally, they stress that they are not trying to imply that such fears are groundless, rather they are arguing that stress and health are complex variables with strong cognitive components.

STUDY 98

Adams, P. R., Adams, G. R., 1984, 'Mount St Helens' ashfall: evidence for a disaster stress reaction', *American Psychologist*, 39, 252–60

Aim

To examine the effects of a natural disaster on a range of stress-related symptoms, such as rates of illness, alcohol abuse, family stress, violence and aggression and mental health. The natural disaster studied here is the Mount St Helens' ashfall, which occurred on 18 May 1980. When the volcano erupted, 57 people were killed, including a researcher studying the volcano's activity.

Method

A natural experiment with repeated measures. The researchers were comparing a variety of measures before and after the Mount St Helens' ashfall.

Participants

The study looked at the town of Othello, Washington (population approximately 5000 people). The town, which is 150 miles away from Mount St Helens, was plunged into total darkness at midday and suffered a serious level of ashfall that took many days to clear.

Procedure

Following the ashfall on 18 May 1980, the researchers collected statistical information from 1 June to 31 December and compared this with the same information for the same months in the previous year. Data was collected on the following:
1) diagnosed illness
2) marital and family problems
3) alcohol abuse
4) rates of aggression and violence
5) general adjustment disorders.

Results

Some of the key results include:
1) Illness – there was an increase of 192 per cent in stress-related illness and increases of over 200 per cent in psychosomatic and mental health disorders.
2) Family problems – there was a decrease of 89 per cent in reports of child abuse and a decrease of 6 per cent in divorce, but an increase of 45 per cent in cases of police-reported domestic violence.
3) Alcohol abuse – there was a general decrease in problems relating to alcohol abuse, drink-driving decreased by 22 per cent, car accidents decreased by 21 per cent and court cases involving driving while intoxicated charges dropped 3 per cent. However, referrals to agencies dealing with alcohol abuse were up 20 per cent and police arrests for violation of the alcohol laws were up 43 per cent.
4) Aggression and violence – in most cases, the data represented an increase in incidents of aggression. Charges of disorderly conduct increased by 10 per cent, vandalism increased by 23 per cent and assaults went up by 27 per cent. However, fewer cases were taken to superior court.
5) General adjustment – mental health appointments increased by 22 per cent and calls to crisis lines increased by 79 per cent.

The results clearly show the extensive stress-reaction effect on the community of Othello.

STUDY 99
Russoniello, C. V., 2002, 'Childhood post-traumatic stress disorder and efforts to cope after Hurricane Floyd', *Behavioral Medicine*, 28, 2, 61–71

Aim	On 15 September 1999, children in eastern California schools were sent home early due to the approaching Hurricane Floyd. Many were evacuated from their homes and many had their homes destroyed by the hurricane. This paper attempts to study the effects of such trauma on a group of schoolchildren who lost their homes. The researchers also attempt to explore the effects of individual characteristics, social environment and coping strategies.
Method	Questionnaire/self-reports.
Participants	218 fourth-grade students, mostly aged nine to ten years. All participants had to have a consent form signed by the parents and the research was approved by the local Institutional Review Board.
Procedure	The research was conducted approximately six months after the hurricane. Researchers used the child version of the Post-Traumatic Stress Reaction Index, which establishes the existence of 20 post-traumatic stress disorder (PTSD) and related symptoms. The researchers also used data collected from KidCope, which measures behavioural and cognitive coping strategies, including distraction, social withdrawal, cognitive restructuring, self-criticism, blaming others, wishful thinking, social support and resignation.
Results	Over 95 per cent of the children reported symptoms of post-traumatic stress disorder, with 71 per cent experiencing moderate to very severe symptoms. Females were experiencing more problems than males and the variable of being flooded at home produced significantly higher levels of symptoms. Most children were using coping strategies (both positive and negative, with the negative strategies being most associated with PTSD), the most commonly used being wishful thinking, cognitive restructuring, social support, distraction, emotional regulation and problem solving. Girls were more likely to use social support than boys and African-American children were more likely to use the strategy of blaming others than the European-American children.
	The researchers conclude this disaster had significant stress-related effects on almost all the children. They also conclude that further research into interventions is essential and suggest that a combination of behavioural medicine and interpersonal techniques would prove to be the most effective.

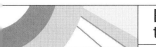

Evaluating research into environmental disaster and technological catastrophe

Ethics
It is difficult to evaluate the ethics of this kind of research. The research by Havenaar *et al.* and by Russoniello clearly raise issues of distress and protection of participants.

Havenaar's research was conducted approximately 15 years after the Chernobyl disaster and this may have meant that any distress caused by the questions may have been less than it might have been had the research been conducted earlier. Indeed, many participants may have been willing to answer these questions as they may have felt that it was important research and they were glad that someone was finally asking them about their feelings. However, it is also possible that people were reminded of events that were extremely distressing or made to think about issues that they had tried to repress in some way. It is important to remember that the participants in this research were adults, whereas the participants in Russoniello's research were young children and this research took place relatively soon after the hurricane. The researcher does state that all parents were asked for consent and that the research was approved. However, this does not detract from the fact that the experience of being questioned may have been very distressing for the children. This is a difficult area for researchers as it is obviously extremely important that such research is conducted. If practical interventions are to be put in place to benefit the victims of such disasters it is also important that the research is conducted relatively quickly. This raises the question of how best to conduct such research. In the studies mentioned so far, the data were collected directly from the people affected and this has obvious strengths, in spite of the potential ethical concerns raised. In contrast to this, the study by Adams and Adams collects data from other sources. They did not question people about their experiences or feelings, but collected data from sources such as hospitals, legal and criminological information and number of calls to helplines. From the point of view of ethics, this resolves the problems identified above as there is no possibility that the research could have added to people's stress.

Type of data collected

As we have identified above, some of this research collected purely quantitative data from 'public' sources and other research collected quantitative and more qualitative data directly from samples of participants. This included the use of Likert scales, as well as formalized psychometric tests such as the Post-Traumatic Stress Reaction Index. These measures have both strengths and weaknesses. On the positive side, Likert items and psychometric tests such as those used by Havenaar *et al.* are easy to administer and analyse. However, they do not give people the option of expanding on their answers; nor do they give the researcher the ability to explore further items in depth. Also they may be prone to demand characteristics; for example, people living near Chernobyl may exaggerate their concerns if they hope that something might be done as a result of the research. Some of the items may be ambiguous or understood differently by different respondents and Likert responses may be difficult to interpret (two people who both feel the same way about an item may give different numbers in response to this item). It is also possible that interpreting the results from these questionnaires may be difficult. For example, the item 'I think that the full extent of the Chernobyl accident is not being told to the public' could be misinterpreted (e.g. people may miss the word 'not' in the statement) and we do not know if the full extent of the Chernobyl accident *is* being told to people. This might mean that people are appearing to be over-anxious when in fact they are not being given the full information. In a similar way, there may be problems with the use of the Post-Traumatic Stress Reaction Index and the KidCope measures used by Russoniello. In contrast, the data collected by Adams and Adams are not prone to demand characteristics as participants are not being asked directly. However, this kind of data could also be inaccurate as there may be more problems than are being reported and there may be other factors that explain these findings.

Level of control/confounding variables

The three studies reported here are all case studies of events. They are pieces of research conducted in response to real-life events and are not conducted in the same way as a laboratory experiment. This gives them some strengths (they have high ecological validity and should be able to be applied directly to helping the people in the affected areas), but it should be remembered that they lack control and it is not easy to generalize their results to other events. The three studies reported here used different designs. The study by Havenaar *et al.* compares people in the affected area with another unaffected area. This is similar to an independent measures (between subjects) design. The researchers claim that the two areas are similar in terms of their socio-economic status and that they both have nuclear power plants. However, there may still be other variables that explain the very different health cognitions that exist in these two populations. These might include other environmental health risks, levels of information, health service availability and so on. In contrast, Adams and Adams use a before-and-after comparison (similar to a repeated measures or within subjects design), which means that they are able to demonstrate a change in behaviours before and after the Mount St Helens' ashfall. This is a powerful research method in environmental psychology, but obviously can only take advantage of the recorded data that is available. It would not be possible to ask people about their behaviours before an event as they would probably not be able to answer these questions very accurately. Finally, Russoniello's research does not have a comparison group, and while this is not a major criticism of the research, it does mean that we cannot compare levels of PTSD in this group of participants with a group who have not experienced this event or who have experienced another event. However, Russoniello does compare variables within the sample and once again demonstrates a gender difference, with females showing a stronger negative reaction to this event (or at least admitting stronger reactions to the researcher). This research also shows differences by race, which is a factor that deserves further exploration.

This research gives you a flavour of the kind of research methods that can be employed when studying environmental disasters and catastrophes. Remember that it is not possible to control all the variables in this kind of research and this should not be seen to detract from its usefulness.

Usefulness

Obviously, it is important that research like this is conducted. These three studies have highlighted a number of different ways in which people respond to environmental disasters and catastrophes and this is extremely useful. This might be applied by researchers who are asked to advise on the possible effects of other disasters or might be applied more directly in the development of resources and services for people in these areas. Although all events are different, there are clearly some common responses and recognition of this is crucial. However, the extraneous variables of gender, race, socio-economic status, educational level, levels of social support and many others mean that predicting possible effects is very difficult indeed.

STUDY 100
Jason, L. A. *et al.*, 1981, 'Territorial behavior on beaches', *The Journal of Social Psychology*, 114, 43–50

Aim	To investigate women's behavioural and emotional reactions to territorial intrusions on a beach.
Method	A combination of observation, experiment and questionnaire methods.
Participants	30 women chosen by opportunity at several beaches in the Chicago area.
Procedure	A male researcher (described as 32 years old and of moderate attractiveness) approached women on a beach. He first asked, 'Do you mind if I sit down?' and then said, 'I am doing a study on beach territoriality – do you mind if I ask you some questions?' Observers also classified the beach as crowded or sparse, estimated the woman's age and rated her attractiveness on a scale of 1–10.

87 per cent of the women approached indicated that the man could sit next to them and all these agreed to answer the questions.

Results	The fact that 87 per cent of the sample allowed a man to invade their territory is significant. It suggests that territory which has not been occupied for very long is highly susceptible to invasion. It also suggests that there are very different expectations surrounding personal space in different territories. Also the women generally reacted positively to the invasion and 61 per cent gave their name and address to the researcher (so they could be sent a copy of the study), indicating a high level of trust and confidence established within a very short space of time. Most of the women indicated that they had dated at least one man whom they had met at the beach (although only 10 per cent had agreed with the statement that they came to the beach to meet men).

STUDY 101
Werner, C. M. *et al.*, 1981, 'Territorial marking in a game arcade', *Journal of Personality and Social Psychology*, 41, 1094–104

Aim

To test the hypothesis that touching can serve territorial functions. It has been well documented that people use physical markers such as books, bags, coats and towels to mark their territory in a variety of locations. Here the authors are investigating the use of touch as a territorial marker in an amusement arcade.

Method

Both observational and experimental methods used.

Participants

78 people playing arcade games. 73 of these were male and only five were female. They were judged to be aged 15–30 years.

Procedure

Only the first part of this study is reported here. This was an observation designed to see if players unfamiliar with the machines they were using would touch machines more than players who were familiar with the machines. Further experimental research was also conducted and the results of this are summarized below.

The researchers hypothesized that novice players would be more likely to touch territory than regular players. A participant was judged to be a novice if they exhibited one of the following behaviours: read the instructions on the wall next to the machine, showed uncertainty about where to put the coin or attempted to put the coin in the wrong place or asked someone to explain the game. Observers then recorded the amount of touching of the machine (excluding necessary manipulation of the controls) that each individual exhibited.

Results

Players unfamiliar with the game touched the machines prior to playing the game, possibly as a way of establishing it as their territory. This behaviour was seen more often in unfamiliar players than in familiar players, although the researchers note that touching was also seen in familiar players. They suggest that where players spend large amounts of time mastering complex games, the machines are perceived as highly desirable territory and this may elicit more territorial behaviour.

Further research reported in this paper also showed that a stranger invading territory (i.e. standing very close to a player) produced high levels of touching behaviour. Also that when a player (actually a confederate) touched the machine, this acted as a deterrent to potential invaders.

The researchers conclude that touching is an effective form of territory marking and, if used in conjunction with other physical markers, would be highly effective.

STUDY 102
Newman, O., 1972, *Defensible Space*, New York: Macmillan, cited in Forsyth, D. R., 1987, *Social Psychology*, Monterey, CA: Brooks Cole

Aim

To investigate the difference between two housing projects based on their levels of defensible space. This research follows Newman's proposals that urban housing projects (large low-cost housing 'estates') should include defensible space. This involves the use of boundaries to give a feeling of control over hallways, lobbies and outside space. It should be possible for residents to have surveillance opportunities and the design of the building should foster positive, protective attitudes. In this study Newman compared two New York housing projects. Van Dyke was built in 1955, including mostly large, 14-storey buildings surrounded by large areas of open space. The Brownsville project was built in 1948 and featured six-storey X-shaped buildings with some three-storey wings. Occupants entered the Brownsville building at the central core where open staircases were located.

Method

A natural experiment.

Procedure

Newman compared the number of crimes committed in each housing project and the number of maintenance jobs required.
    These were broken down as follows:
    Crime – felonies, misdemeanours and offences, robberies, malicious mischief and other crimes.
    Maintenance jobs – maintenance jobs other than glass repair, number of full-time maintenance staff required and number of elevator breakdowns per month.

Results

The results show a striking difference between the two projects. Newman reports a total of 1189 crimes in the Van Dyke project compared with 790 in the Brownsville project. This included 92 robberies in the Van Dyke project and only 24 in the Brownsville project. The total number of maintenance jobs in the Van Dyke project was 3301, compared to a lower figure of 2376 in the Brownsville project.
    Newman concludes that the Brownsville project was much more defensible than the Van Dyke project. In particular, he claims that this is due to the fact that the Brownsville project had entrances used by smaller numbers of people and that these entrances could be seen from dozens of windows. This has the effect of making people feel more territorial about the communal space. In this project, people let their children play in the hallways and often left their doors open to 'keep an eye on the place'. As well as the lower crime and maintenance rates, this housing project was also associated with more positive relationships between neighbours and less negative attitudes towards the police.

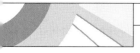

Evaluating research into personal space and territory

Ecological validity/application to real life

Ecological validity is high in all three studies as all were conducted in real-life situations. Application to everyday life is slightly different, however. The study by Jason *et al.* strongly suggests that there are different sorts of territories and that people react differently to their invasion. This study suggests that a beach seems to be a place where people are often actually asking for their territory to be invaded. If you think about what people wear on the beach they are clearly giving out certain signals! This would mean that you should not apply the results of research in a situation such as a beach to another situation such as a library or a medical setting. The study by Werner *et al.* also has high ecological validity as it was mainly conducted as an observation in a public place, with people unaware that they were being observed. Even the experimental manipulations were not such that the situation was made unnatural. Finally, Newman's research compared two real housing projects and hence has extremely high ecological validity.

Levels of control/confounding variables

There are a number of other variables that might have contributed to the results of the research. In particular, the researcher himself could be described as a confounding variable in Jason *et al.*'s research. The researcher was male, 32 and described as being of 'moderate attractiveness'. He was approaching females who were alone on a beach. If the same researcher had invaded a male's territory, the results may have been somewhat different. Similarly, if the researcher had been female or an older less attractive male, the female participants may have acted very differently. In research like this, the personal characteristics of the researcher need to be taken into account and perhaps research like this should be replicated with a different researcher in order to examine the effect. In the research by Werner *et al.*, the conclusion is that touching the machines is a form of territory marking and although this is most likely the case, these behaviours may also have different functions or stem from different causes. Novice players may be less confident people generally or have different personality characteristics to those who regularly play arcade games and this may contribute to different forms of non-verbal behaviour. The research by Newman compares just two housing projects and there may be other differences between them apart from their design. They may be in different areas, nearer to or further away from other housing projects, easier to get to, house different people, have different age profiles and so on. Control over all these variables is obviously impossible in this sort of research, but it needs to be borne in mind.

Ethics/ethical implications

The studies reported in this section do not raise serious ethical issues, although there are some minor issues with the two studies into territorial behaviour and an issue of ethical implications with Newman's research. Observations in public places are not considered unethical and both a beach and a games arcade could be considered public spaces. However, Werner *et al.* also conducted some experimental research in the games arcade without the knowledge or consent of his participants. It is difficult to imagine any negative consequences of this research, but strictly speaking you should not conduct experimental research on participants without their consent. The experimenter in the Jason *et al.* study approached women and asked to sit down before explaining that he was conducting research. Some women may have felt intimidated by this approach and indeed 13 per cent did not agree that he could sit down. Again, these are very minor issues, but they highlight the difficulties of conducting research on these kinds of topics without infringing ethical guidelines at all. Finally, Newman's research does not raise any ethical issues as he did no more than collect data on crimes and maintenance jobs in each housing project. However, there are ethical implications to this kind of research. If indeed there are other factors responsible for the different levels of crime found in each housing project, then to publish a study that concluded that this was due to the design of the buildings would be unwise and could have a number of implications. People might be put off living in one project; those living in the Van Dyke project may become scapegoats; and future designs may lay too much emphasis on design features at the expense of other factors. It could be argued that research like Newman's comes under the heading of 'socially sensitive research' and researchers need to consider the implications of publication very carefully indeed.

Usefulness

Despite the points made above, it can be argued that Newman's research is extremely useful. His work has had a major impact on the way buildings are designed and also has many useful suggestions to make for environmental crime prevention. Better lighting, clearly defined territory and so on have all proved highly effective in reducing crime rates. The other two pieces of research do not have the same levels of practical application, but it could be argued that both increase our understanding of territorial behaviour significantly. Jason *et al.*'s research demonstrates that there are very different forms of territory and invasion in one situation is not experienced as invasion in another. Werner *et al.* demonstrated that there are forms of territorial marking other than placing possessions as markers or boundaries and that touching of territory is a highly effective form of territorial marking.

ENVIRONMENT
Architecture and behaviour

STUDY 103
Spencer, C., Woolley, H., 2000, 'Children and the city: a summary of recent environmental psychology research', *Child: Care, Health and Development*, 26, 3, 181–98

Aim

To review recent environmental psychology research that focuses on children's needs and experiences of towns and cities. The researchers start from the premise that children's needs are ignored by those who plan and manage urban areas.

Method

A review.

Procedure

The researchers have not conducted all the research reported here, but are bringing together research on a wide variety of issues relating to children in urban areas. These include place attachments, the affordances (what the environment offers in a psycho-social sense) of towns and cities for well-being and development, social and physical dangers, children's favourite places and exploration and its role in social and cognitive development. In this summary only a selection of the key findings are presented.

Results

1) Children's needs are not taken into account. Most urban planning/design reflects adult needs and values. This has the effect of making children an 'out-group' in urban areas. The researchers cite a study by Sebba (1991), who found that adults almost always identified their favourite childhood place as an outdoor place without adult supervision and Sebba's research implies that this may have changed with successive generations. Children aged 10–12 years who were interviewed by the authors were unhappy with many of the public spaces available to them and commented on the high levels of vandalism, litter and graffiti. Gaster (1991), using a combination of contemporary and retrospective data, found that over three generations urban space for children has been gradually 'eroded', with informal areas being replaced with formal directed play areas.

2) Cities are perceived as becoming more dangerous and there are several studies mentioned which demonstrate how fears of crime, kidnapping and assault are on the increase. In particular, a study by Bjorklid (1994) identifies the increase in 'traffic environmental stress' and cites this as leading to increased social isolation in urban areas. It is not just adults who show an increased anxiety about all these issues; children, too, are very aware of danger spots in terms of crime and this has a powerful effect on their use of urban areas. Children also show a sophisticated understanding of pollution and its effects.

3) Overall the results paint a picture of children ignored by planners and excluded from using many areas of towns and cities. If there are no designated areas for children, and public areas are not child-friendly, problems will arise. Either

children will use inappropriate spaces (increasing the risk of the development of antisocial activities) or they will become more and more socially isolated. As parents become more and more anxious about the dangers facing children, they will be more and more likely to keep their children in. This may have some significant effects on identity development if children have no outside space that they can use away from parental supervision. The authors quote Buss (1995) as saying: 'at an age when they should be individuating from their parents, forging an autonomous identity, negotiating relationships with peers [they are] instead grappling with everyday survival issues such as "Will I be shot today?"'

4) Finally, the authors report on a number of ways in which children can become involved in environmental planning. These include action-research to include children's voices in environmental planning as well as environmental education. Interestingly, this review points out that curriculum reforms in the UK have virtually removed environmental education from British schools.

STUDY 104
Baum, A., Davis, G., 1980, 'Reducing the stress of high-density living: an architectural intervention', *Journal of Personality and Social Psychology*, 38, 471–81

Aim

To investigate the effects of an architectural intervention on residential crowding.

It has been well documented that high-density shared housing is associated with negative psychosocial effects. In this paper, the researchers attempt to manipulate density experimentally through the building of a dividing wall to separate previously high-density shared housing into two.

Method

This research involved surveys, observations and experimental procedures.

Participants

Undergraduate female students in a US university. There were three conditions:
1) a long corridor floor housing 40 students
2) a short corridor floor housing three groups of 20 students
3) an altered long corridor floor, which had been separated into two groups of 20 students.

Procedure

All participants were asked to complete a questionnaire on the day they moved in and then again after five weeks and after 12 weeks. These assessed feelings about college, dormitory life, other students and how they spent their time. Some of the key questions asked participants to rate (on Likert scales) how crowded, hectic and predictable dormitory life was, success at controlling social interactions and control of space in the dormitory. Observations were conducted between the third and the fourteenth weeks, but always between 10 and 11 p.m. The observer noted the number of social interactions taking place as well as the number of bedroom doors open. Finally, an experiment was conducted. Participants were tested one at a time and spent some time 'waiting' with a confederate. Social interaction with the confederate was observed. Then participants were asked to complete a questionnaire (on general issues such as sleep and eating patterns, levels of control felt over the situation and so on). Then the participant was shown into another room and asked to solve a series of 12 anagrams.

Results

Some of the most important results include: there was evidence of higher stress and control-related problems among residents of the long corridor. Long corridor residents also reported less small group interaction, fewer friends made and less control over social experiences. These effects were reduced by the architectural intervention described above. By the sixth week of observation, less social interaction was observed in the long corridor than in the other two environments, and fewer bedroom doors were left open. Finally, the laboratory research suggested similar findings: less interaction from the long corridor residents (they sat further away, made less eye contact and reported feeling more uncomfortable) and less time spent trying to solve anagrams.

The researchers conclude that the architectural intervention was a success, resulting in greater positive social interaction, more group development, a higher sense of control and less social withdrawal.

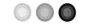

STUDY 105
Keeley, R. M., Edney, J. J., 1983, 'Model house design for privacy, security and social interaction', *The Journal of Social Psychology*, 119, 219–28

Aim
To evaluate house designs produced by undergraduate students. The students were asked to design houses that would promote either privacy, security or social interaction for the occupants. Designs produced by males, females and mixed pairs were also compared.

Method
A laboratory-based experiment with repeated measures (three different conditions). Also compared the naturally occurring variable of gender.

Participants
Undergraduate students enrolled for a course called Environmental Design. 20 males worked independently, 20 females worked independently and 20 male–female pairs worked together.

Procedure
Each individual or pair was asked to build three model houses, one each for privacy, security and social interaction (order was counterbalanced). They were provided with standard model-building equipment and also transferred the design for their house on to paper once completed. Plans were then assessed on a number of features, including: number and size of rooms, number of communal spaces, number of bedrooms adjoining each other, number of rooms with/without outside walls, number of interior and exterior openings, number of rooms leading off a common space, number of corridors, shape of house, symmetry of design, outside features and so on.

Results
Overall, houses built for privacy had more (smaller) rooms, more corridor space, more interior doors and more external wall surfaces (often as participants 'tacked' rooms on to the side of the house). Houses built for security were the smallest, possibly to keep the occupants close together to give a sense of security or to make the defensible space as small as possible. Further, houses built for security had the smallest number of bedrooms with outside walls. Finally, houses built for social interaction had the greatest visibility within the interior (open-plan designs), the largest proportion of communal space and, interestingly, were most likely to include concave curved walls. These are thought to promote social interaction in the way that round tables do – everyone is equidistant from everyone else and therefore equally involved, while square rooms (or tables) have corners that allow people to isolate themselves.

There were also significant sex differences in house design. Females designed smaller models than males, had higher ratios of communal areas to bedroom space, more exterior walls, less symmetry in their models and were rated as producing the more original designs. The researchers conclude that they have identified some useful design heuristics.

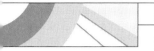

Evaluating research into architecture and behaviour

Research methods

There are a range of research methods used in these studies. The research by Spencer and Woolley is a review article, which means that the researchers are not simply reporting on one piece of research that they have conducted (although they do include their own research), but bringing together numerous pieces of research on related areas. This is a valuable contribution to research as it shows how a number of variables interact to produce effects, in contrast to the other experimental studies, which focus on the effect of one variable at a time. It is also useful to be able to see how a relatively new area of research is developing, and one of the striking features of this review article is the fact that it includes research from a number of different areas of the world. Baum and Davis conducted an experimental study looking at the variable of 'architectural intervention', in this case, the dividing up of large communal student accommodation into smaller units. This research has a number of controls, including questionnaires given at set times, some controlled experimental research and observations. However, as it is an experimental study it focuses on just one variable and there may be a number of factors which interact to produce the effects described. Finally, Keeley and Edney used a simulation procedure in their experiment and while this would give their experiment high levels of control there may be some issues related to ecological validity.

Ecological validity/application to real life

The research by Baum and Davis is conducted in student accommodation. The students were unaware that the alterations that had been made to their living accommodation were being studied and hence there would be reduced demand characteristics in this research. This study has high ecological validity as it was conducted in a real-life environment, although you could argue that it would be difficult to generalize these results to anything other than student accommodation.

The experimental study included by Baum and Davis looking at levels of social interaction in a controlled environment and time spent solving anagrams may have lower ecological validity; one might be able to question the conclusion that high-density living causes withdrawal from social interaction had this been the only way in which this had been measured. The study by Keeley and Edney has very low ecological validity as it studied house design through the building of small-scale cardboard models. They have identified some useful design heuristics, although (as the authors note themselves) some real-world research needs to be conducted before any strong conclusions can be drawn.

Sampling

Baum and Davis studied US undergraduate students. 140 female students were included in this research. There are a number of issues arising from this sample. You could consider the possibility for generalization to other samples. Does research conducted with students tell us anything about other groups? When you go to university you may expect that you will live in relatively high-density accommodation, you may have another home to go to in the holidays, you are aware that this is short-term accommodation and so on. It would be difficult to suggest that people living long-term in this level of high-density accommodation would respond in the same way. Arguably, their responses would be more extreme, as we have seen in the 'Density and crowding' section of this chapter, but there may also be cultural issues here. Housing expectations differ across the world; what in a western society may be regarded as crowded may be seen very differently in other countries. Finally, the gender issue needs to be considered once again. We have seen in numerous pieces of research in this chapter that males and females respond differently to environmental stressors. This means that we should be cautious about interpreting results from female-only samples as applying equally to males. Keeley and Edney also used US undergraduate students for their research, although this sample differs in two important respects: first, they used equal numbers of males and females (and compared this variable) and second, the students were all enrolled on a course called Environmental Design. This is clearly an interesting sample to use, with the advantage that they would have experience of model building etc., but the results from this sample may not be representative of other populations, either within the USA or in other cultures. Finally, this research once again demonstrates a difference in the ways that males and females interact with their environment.

Usefulness

There are many useful applications of the research described here. The review article brings together a range of different studies and draws some useful general conclusions. The authors highlight the necessity for children's needs to be taken into account in planning and development processes as well as the need for good environmental education. The research highlights the potential psychological effect of living in urban areas with no safe places for children, increasing pollution levels, fear and crime. It may be that at present the useful application of this review is simply to highlight the area as requiring further research, but longer term such research may have very many practical applications, both for planners and educators and for those working in the mental health professions.

Baum and Davis's research has many useful applications for those designing accommodation for students. It is clear that high-density accommodation can have negative health effects, which, in turn, could impact on students' performance. If costs allowed, it would be sensible for university management to put a maximum figure on shared accommodation. However, whether these results apply equally to male students or to other types of housing are less clear. Finally, Keeley and Edney's study highlights the need for planners to determine the most important needs for occupants of new houses. Different design features need to be incorporated for security, privacy or social interaction. Hence houses designed for the elderly may concentrate on security aspects, while houses designed for young families would concentrate on space for social interaction. The finding that males and females design different kinds of space is also a useful one and deserves further exploration.

STUDY 106
Gwinn, H. M. *et al.*, 2002, 'Do landmarks help or hinder women in route learning?', *Perceptual and Motor Skills*, 95, 713–18

| Aim | Several research studies have documented that men are able to learn routes faster and with fewer errors than women, whereas women are able to recall more landmarks along the route. This study aims to see if the use of landmarks will help or hinder women when they learn a route. |

Aim

Several research studies have documented that men are able to learn routes faster and with fewer errors than women, whereas women are able to recall more landmarks along the route. This study aims to see if the use of landmarks will help or hinder women when they learn a route.

Method

An experiment with independent measures (two conditions) and also comparing the naturally occurring variable of gender.

Participants

47 female and 37 male undergraduate students, who were recruited for a 'map tracing' experiment and received extra course credits for participation.

Procedure

Participants were randomly assigned to one of two conditions, either learning a route on a map with landmarks (schools, rivers, named buildings etc.) or learning the same route on a map with no landmarks (road outlines only). They were shown the map, told which direction was north and then shown the route followed by a school bus. The route consisted of 11 left turns and nine right turns. Participants were shown once and then asked to trace the route on a map. Mistakes were immediately corrected and each participant continued until they had traced the route correctly on two consecutive attempts. The time it took to reach this point was recorded, as were the total number of trials and the number of errors made.

Results

Men did better than women in the landmark condition but there was no significant difference in the no-landmark condition. Men learned the route faster and more accurately when landmarks were present, but women's performance was not affected by the presence or absence of landmarks. This suggests that men and women use landmarks differently when learning routes and that landmarks may in fact interfere with women's learning of routes.

STUDY 107
Bryant, K. J., 1982, 'Personality correlates of sense of direction and geographical orientation', *Journal of Personality and Social Psychology*, 41, 6, 1318–24

Aim

The researchers point out that it is well known that individuals' self-reports of their sense of direction accurately predict their ability to point to unseen familiar locations. These factors also correlate with self-reports of anxiety about getting lost, concern over following new directions, reading maps and so on. In this study the researchers are looking for personality correlates of geographical orientation. They are predicting a correlation between self-reported sense of direction, anxiety about getting lost, visuo-spatial skills and personality variables, with a behavioural measure of pointing accuracy.

Method

A natural experiment comparing the naturally occurring variable of gender. Questionnaires and skills tests used to measure sense of direction and geographical orientation.

Participants

85 undergraduate students from the University of California (45 female, 40 male), who had lived on campus for 20 weeks or more.

Procedure

Participants completed a number of tasks:
1) Sense of Direction questionnaire – measured items such as self-estimates of spatial ability, responses to disorientation and ability to give and follow directions
2) a paper-and-pencil pointing task – participants had to imagine themselves at various points on campus and describe the view that they would have; they were then given a drawing of a circle showing the direction in which they were facing and asked to mark the direction of nine target locations
3) Mental Rotations Test – measures ability to represent spatial relationships internally
4) California Psychological Inventory – assesses a variety of psychological dimensions to do with interpersonal behaviour and social interaction – these include flexibility, sociability, self-acceptance, capacity for status (defined as personal qualities and attributes that underlie and lead to the attainment of status and symbols of success) and intellectual efficiency.

Results

Individuals' self-reports of their sense of direction accurately predicted their pointing scores. Generally, males' self-reports were higher than those of females and males did better on the pointing task. The results showed that personality scores also contributed to ability in pointing tasks; in particular, sociability, self-acceptance and capacity for status appeared to be crucial dispositions in the acquisition and accuracy of mental representations of the environment. Overall these results suggest that different personalities interact with their environment in different ways and this has a significant effect on the environmental representations that they form.

> **STUDY 108**
> Evans, G. *et al.*, 1980, 'Cognitive mapping and architecture', *Journal of Applied Psychology*,
> 65, 474–8

Aim

To test the effects of colour-coding of a building's interior on orientation.

Method

An experiment (independent variable was whether the building was colour-coded or not).

Participants

Two groups of seven undergraduate students at the University of California. They were told that the aim of the research was to assess opinions about building architecture.

Procedure

All participants were given an individual tour of either a colour-coded or a non-colour-coded unfamiliar building. They were then asked to walk in the most direct route to three different locations within the building. If they did not find the required location within five minutes, the experimenter would collect them and reassure them that this was a very difficult task.

Results

Participants in the colour-coded condition made fewer errors (deviations from the shortest route) in the finding-the-way task and could identify locations on plans more accurately. The researchers conclude that colour-coding of the interior of large institutional buildings can be highly effective and suggest that these effects may be of particular benefit to the elderly and to institutionalized mental patients or in buildings where the majority of users will not visit often enough to become familiar with the layout of the building.

Evaluating research into environmental cognition

Ecological validity

The research by Gwinn *et al.* has low ecological validity. Participants were asked to learn a route on a map and then trace the route with their finger on the same map. This is not measuring route-learning in an ecologically valid way. In real life you might learn a map from paper, but your learning would be tested when you actually tried to find your way from one place to another. Landmarks may operate in different ways in the real world than on maps and it may be that some participants would be able to use the landmarks to help them in the real world even though they did not help in the experimental situation. In a similar way, the study by Bryant used a paper-and-pencil pointing task, which may give different results to actually asking people to point in the correct direction in the real world. However, if the research is investigating environmental representations (rather than finding the way) then this is a valid way of assessing the internal representations that the students have. Finally, the research by Evans *et al.* has the highest ecological validity. In this study participants were shown round a building and then asked to find certain locations. This has high ecological validity as they are finding their way around a real building.

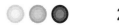

Gender differences

Once again, the research described in this section raises the issues of gender differences. Gwinn et al.'s research confirms other findings that men generally are better at route learning. However, the landmark versus no-landmark variable shows that women were not affected by the presence of landmarks. Other research shows that women are more likely than men to remember landmarks along routes and this finding may be a result of the low ecological validity discussed above. Landmarks on maps may not have the same impact as landmarks in the real world.

Bryant's study also confirms gender differences in environmental cognition. Bryant found that men rated their sense of direction more highly than women did and also did better on the pointing task.

Sampling

As well as the gender issue described above, there are other issues related to sampling raised by this research. First, all three studies use undergraduate students and there are problems in generalizing this research to other groups. It may be that undergraduates have different ways of interacting with their environments that might affect these results. For example, in the research by Bryant, all the undergraduates had lived on campus for 20 weeks or more. Perhaps due to social factors, males explore their environments more than females do and the difference in pointing ability is simply a difference in how familiar the landmarks were. A campus is a closed environment and it would be interesting to see if the same differences were found in a small town or even a large city. Second, the undergraduates recruited for Gwinn et al.'s study were awarded course credits and this may have influenced their behaviour. Perhaps they would be very keen to show that they could do well and again this may reduce the generalizability of the findings. Finally, the sample size in Evans et al.'s research is small (only 14 undergraduates) and it is difficult to draw strong conclusions about the effects of colour on location finding from such a small group.

Usefulness

There are several useful applications of this research. Perhaps the most useful application comes from Evans et al., who has demonstrated that the use of colour-coding in buildings can help people negotiate them. This might have particular benefits for young children in large unfamiliar school buildings, the elderly and those with memory-related mental health problems or in buildings such as hospitals that have large numbers of infrequent visitors. This is a particularly useful application as it would be relatively easy and inexpensive to apply. Gwinn et al.'s research adds to the large body of research stating that maps are easier for men to understand than women. This could be applied to state that there is a need to investigate how women learn routes and how maps could be designed to reflect this type of cognition. The useful application of Bryant's research is not immediately obvious, but it is useful to understand how combinations of variables interact and Bryant demonstrates clearly that different types of personalities have very different internal representations of their world.

See also...	

Studies 6, 7, 55, 80 and 82.

Section 5
SPORT

SPORT
Personality and sport

STUDY 109
Morgan, W. P., O'Connor, P. J., Sparling, B. P., Rate, R. R., 1987, 'Psychological characterization of the elite female distance runner', *International Journal of Sports Medicine*, 8, 124–31

Aim

The initial aim was to identify psychological differences between elite and non-elite runners. The researchers went on to compare the sample as a whole with population averages in order to identify differences.

Method

Questionnaires and interviews.

Participants

The sample comprised 27 volunteers, including 15 elite and 12 non-elite distance runners. The runners' distances ranged from 1500m to marathons. The non-elite runners initially formed the control group.

Procedure

Participants signed an informed consent document. They were told that the results would be treated confidentially, that they would remain anonymous and that they were free to discontinue involvement at any point.

Participants completed a series of psychological questionnaires and a 24-hour history during the first evening. The questionnaires included:
1) Eysenck's Personality Questionnaire
2) Profile of Mood States
3) State-Trait Anxiety Inventory
4) Body Awareness Scale.

The 24-hour history involved a questionnaire focusing on the individual's general state of well-being, as well as exercise and sleep patterns over the previous 24 hours. It was used as a means of identifying runners who were experiencing problems of any kind, which might influence the psychological test results.

A structured interview was also carried out with each participant where specific topics were addressed, including:
1) motivation (intrinsic and extrinsic)
2) cognitive strategies
3) race strategies
4) training volume
5) staleness
6) pre-competition arousal.

Ratings of perceived exertion were also obtained during a sub-maximal run on a treadmill.

Results

Questionnaires – initial analysis of the results of the questionnaires showed that there were no significant differences between the elite and non-elite groups; Morgan *et al.* then made the decision to combine the data from the two groups and compare the combined results with population averages. Results from the POMS showed that the combined group possessed the 'iceberg profile' typical of elite athletes, scoring lower than the population average on negative moods (such as tension, depression, anger) and significantly higher on vigour. Analysis of the EPQ showed that the group was slightly more extroverted and stable than the general population. The STAI analysis showed that state and trait anxiety scores in the group did not differ from published norms.

Interview – motivation for initial involvement and for continuing to train and compete was significantly higher for the intrinsic category than the extrinsic category. There was a significant difference in the proportion of runners who employed associative attentional strategies (directing attention internally) (56 per cent) compared to disassociative strategies (directing attention externally) (22 per cent) during competition, but this relationship was reversed during training. Results of the BAS questionnaire showed that the group's arousal level increased significantly in the pre-competition setting; however, significant individual differences were found between individual arousal levels (supporting the view that a Zone of Optimal Functioning exists for each individual). During the interview each runner was asked whether they had experienced staleness in the past (a condition thought to be due to over-training); results showed that 48 per cent had experienced staleness and that the incidence of staleness was higher in the elite runners.

STUDY 110

Williams, L. T. R., Parkin, W. A., 1980, 'Personality factor profiles of three hockey groups', *International Journal of Sports Psychology*, 11, 113–20

| Aim | To test a sample of field hockey players at three different performance levels in order to identify personality differences between the groups. |

| Method | A questionnaire. |

| Participants | The sample comprised 85 male hockey players, including 18 internationals (elite), 34 nationals and 33 club players (non-elite). |

| Procedure | Form A of the 16PF Personality Questionnaire (Cattell) was administered to all participants. |

| Results | Analysis of the 16PF questionnaires showed several differences between the groups. The international group had significantly different personality profiles to the club group. The national group's profiles were not significantly distinguishable from the other two groups, but were more similar to the international group. The personality factors which contributed most significantly to the difference between the elite group and the others included confidence, intelligence, emotional stability and tough-mindedness. These results were compared with those of previous similar studies and it was found that similar personality factors distinguished the elite performers from the non-elite (see Kroll & Krenshaw, 1970 – football players, Williams, 1975 – rowers). |

Evaluating research into personality and sport

Sampling

There are two main issues regarding the sample in the Morgan *et al.* study, namely, the size and selection method. The sample comprised 27 in total, initially divided into two groups of 15 and 12. This is a very small sample, which consequently has a greater potential for bias as individual differences between participants will have a greater impact on overall results in a small sample. It is also more difficult to achieve significant results from a small sample (which may have contributed to the non-significant results in the initial stages of the study). The participants are also all female and all distance runners, which limits the groups that the results can be generalized to. The sampling method used was self-selection (volunteers), which again creates the potential for bias as volunteers are thought to be atypical of the general population. The ideal sampling method is random sampling, which causes the least bias but is often difficult to achieve.

The sample used in the Williams and Parkin study is larger and includes different ability levels. However, they are all male hockey players, so the results are not easily generalized to females or participants in other sports.

Use of questionnaires

There are various problems with the use of questionnaires, including their validity and reliability. The validity problem stems from the lack of universally agreed definitions of terms such as personality itself, as well as many of the personality factors the test claims to be measuring. The reliability of the 16PF has been questioned by Cattell himself, as he acknowledges that individual responses and scores may vary according to mood, motivation and situational factors.

Other problems include the suggestion that only partial information is collected by questionnaires and that the participants may show a social desirability bias by answering in such a way as to show themselves in the best light rather than answering truthfully.

Use of interviews

The study by Morgan *et al.* used interviews as well as questionnaires to gather data. The problems with interviews include the partial collection of data or the misinterpretation of that data. Demand characteristics may be shown where, because they are participating in research, participants answer in the way they think is expected of them. They may also give socially desirable answers. There may also be interviewer effects, where factors about the interviewer – such as age, gender, ethnic group, appearance – can have an effect on the interviewee. Interviews are also time-consuming and require specific skills on the part of the interviewer in order to gain the maximum amount of relevant information from participants.

Ethics

Personality testing is a sensitive process and testers should not probe beyond what is necessary. The athlete's permission must be given and the full details of what is involved and the purpose of the test must be explained. Results should remain confidential and permission should be gained before giving the results to anyone else. Finally, the tester should be qualified to administer the test and interpret the results. Most of these ethical issues were addressed in the Morgan *et al.* study where they gained informed consent, assured anonymity and confidentiality of information and allowed withdrawal at any point.

Individual and situational explanations

These studies use only the 16PF and the EPQ to measure personality, with questionnaires based on the Trait Approach to personality. This approach adopts an individual explanation, suggesting that personality consists of a set of stable characteristics which are not greatly affected by situational factors. Other approaches suggest that personality is situational or is influenced by an interaction between traits and situation. These research studies give little consideration to situational influences on personality.

SPORT
Aggression in sport

STUDY 111
Bandura, A., Ross, D., Ross, S., 1961, 'Transmission of aggression through imitation of aggressive models', *Journal of Abnormal and Social Psychology*, 63, 375–82

Aim	

To demonstrate that children will imitate aggressive behaviour that they have witnessed in an adult.

Method	

A laboratory experiment.

Participants	

72 children (36 boys, 36 girls), aged 37–69 months. One male adult and one female adult acted as the models.

Procedure	

The experiment had three main conditions: a control group, an aggressive model condition and a non-aggressive model condition. In the aggressive and non-aggressive model conditions the children observed an adult playing with a set of children's toys. These groups were further subdivided by the gender of the children and the gender of the adult model. Hence the groups were as follows:
1) Control group (n = 24)
2) Aggressive model condition (n = 24)
   a. boys with same-sex model (n = 6)
   b. boys with opposite-sex model (n = 6)
   c. girls with same-sex model (n = 6)
   d. girls with opposite-sex model (n = 6)
3) Non-aggressive model condition (n = 24)
   a. boys with same-sex model (n = 6)
   b. boys with opposite-sex model (n = 6)
   c. girls with same-sex model (n = 6)
   d. girls with opposite-sex model (n = 6).

The children were all pre-tested and assessed for aggressiveness so that all groups could be matched in terms of how aggressive the children initially were. The children were all tested individually. The experiment consisted of three stages:

Stage 1 – the child was put in the corner of a room with a set of interesting activities to complete. The adult model went to the opposite corner of the room and began playing with a set of children's toys, including a mallet and a 5-foot Bobo doll. In the non-aggressive condition, the adult played in a quiet, subdued manner, ignoring the Bobo, while in the aggressive condition, the adult played in a distinctively aggressive manner with the doll.

Stage 2 – the child was subjected to 'mild aggression arousal' by being taken to a room with attractive toys and, after starting to play with them, being told that they were the experimenter's best toys that he was reserving for other children.

Stage 3 – the child was taken to a room which contained a variety of both aggressive and non-aggressive toys, including a 3-foot Bobo doll and a mallet.

The child was observed playing with the toys for 20 minutes through a one-way mirror. The observers recorded three measures of imitation, including:
1) imitations of physical aggression
2) imitations of verbal aggression
3) imitations of non-aggressive verbal responses.

Results

The children in the aggressive conditions performed more aggressive acts than those in the non-aggressive conditions. Boys performed more aggressive acts than girls. Boys in the aggressive conditions showed more aggression if the model was male. Girls in the aggressive conditions showed more physical aggression if the model was male, but more verbal aggression if the model was female.

In a later experiment using the same format (Bandura, 1965) the children in the aggressive conditions were divided into three groups following stage 2 of the experiment. The first went straight into the playroom, a second group saw the model being rewarded for their aggressiveness and a third group saw the model being punished. The results of this study showed that the children who saw the model being punished for aggression displayed significantly less aggression themselves than those who saw the model being rewarded or those who witnessed no consequences.

STUDY 112
Berkowitz, L., LePage, A., 1967, 'Weapons as aggression-eliciting stimuli', *Journal of Personality and Social Psychology*, 7, 202–7

Aim	

To investigate the hypothesis that stimuli commonly associated with aggression can elicit aggressive responses from people ready to act aggressively.

Method	

A laboratory experiment.

Participants	

100 male psychology students who volunteered in order to gain points towards their final grade.

Procedure	

Participants were told that they would be involved in an experiment on the effects of stress on problem solving. They each worked with a partner who was introduced as a fellow participant, but who was in fact a confederate of the experimenter (referred to as the 'target'). Both were asked to work out the solution to a problem.

Participants were then told that their partner would be evaluating their solution by giving them between one and ten mild electric shocks – one for a good solution, ten for a poor solution (the number of shocks was actually decided by the experimenter and consisted of either one shock, referred to as the 'non-angered condition', or seven shocks, referred to as the 'angered condition').

Participants were then asked to evaluate the target's solution by giving them between one and ten electric shocks. In fact, no shocks were given as the machine was bogus, but researchers were able to measure the participant's level of aggression by counting the number of shocks they believed they were administering. While the participant carried out their evaluation there were sometimes objects present in the room, including a badminton racket and shuttlecock or a shotgun and revolver, which were either described as belonging to their partner or to someone else.

In total there were seven conditions in this experiment:
1) angered, no objects present
2) non-angered, no objects present
3) angered, unassociated weapons present
4) non-angered, unassociated weapons present
5) angered, associated weapons present
6) non-angered, associated weapons present
7) angered, badminton racket present.

The dependent variable was measured by the number of shocks given to the target, the duration of those shocks and self-ratings of mood before and after shocking the target.

Results	

The greatest number of shocks was given by the angered participants in the presence of weapons. More shocks were given when the weapons were associated with the target, but not significantly more. Analysis of mood scales after initial shocks showed that angered participants were significantly more angry and sad than non-angered participants. There was no significant change in mood seen in participants before and after they had shocked the target.

Mean number of shocks given in each condition:

Condition	Shocks received	
	1 ('non-angered')	7 ('angered')
Associated weapons	2.60	6.07
Unassociated weapons	2.20	5.67
No objects	3.07	4.67
Badminton racket	—	4.60

STUDY 113
Daniels, K., Thornton, E. W., 1990, 'An analysis of the relationship between hostility and training in the martial arts', *Journal of Sports Sciences*, 8, 95–101

Aim

To test how martial artists compared with participants in other sports in their levels of hostility, and to establish whether length of martial arts training appeared to increase or decrease hostility.

Method

A questionnaire.

Participants

90 students from Liverpool University, comprising five groups, each of 18 participants:
1) members of the karate club
2) members of the jiu-jitsu club
3) members of the rugby club
4) members of the badminton club
5) non-athletes.

Procedure

The hostility of each group was measured using a modernized version of the Buss-Durkee Hostility Inventory, developed in 1957. The questionnaire comprised 32 questions which measured three types of hostility:
1) assaultive (violent)
2) indirect (tantrums and destructive behaviour)
3) verbal.
Groups 1–4 completed the questionnaire at training sessions; group 5 completed it in their rooms.

Results

No significant differences were found between the hostility of the five groups. Beginners in martial arts showed higher levels of hostility than other athletes. Experienced martial artists showed lower levels of hostility than other athletes. Analysis of the sub-scales showed that assaultive hostility declined significantly with length of martial arts training, whereas indirect hostility increased slightly.

Evaluating research into aggression in sport

Ethics
Research involving aggression is likely to have ethical problems. Both the Bandura *et al.* and the Berkowitz and LePage studies can be considered unethical as they provide the opportunity for participants to display aggression. In the Bandura *et al.* study the participants were young children and there is no mention of parental consent being given. The children were exposed to an aggressive adult, which may have been distressing; they were aroused by having toys taken away from them and were then given the opportunity to imitate the aggression. The possibility of long-term harm to these children is a cause for concern in this study. In the Berkowitz and LePage study the participants were angered by being given electric shocks and

were then allowed to vent their anger on another person. In contrast, the Daniels and Thornton study could be considered to be an ethical study. Questionnaire studies typically have fewer ethical problems than experimental research as manipulation of behaviour is less likely.

Ecological validity

Both the Bandura *et al.* and the Berkowitz and LePage studies are laboratory experiments, which typically have low ecological validity. In both studies the situations that the participants were put into were highly artificial and bear little relation to everyday life. As such it is questionable whether these studies actually tell us anything about real-life aggression.

Nature/nurture debate

The Bandura *et al.* study provides some evidence that aggression can be learned through observation and imitation, suggesting a nurture explanation. However, the Daniels and Thornton study provides some support for an alternative explanation. The Instinct Approach suggests that we are naturally aggressive and that this aggression builds up inside us and requires some outlet. A legitimate outlet can be provided by sport, and so participation in sport should reduce aggression, as shown by Daniels and Thornton.

Usefulness/practical applications

As much sport includes aggression, research which tells us more about the causes of aggression, the conditions under which it is most likely to occur and how it can be controlled or reduced is likely to be useful. The Bandura *et al.* study suggests that aggression can be learned through observation and imitation. This has particular relevance for sport as sport provides many role models, particularly for children. The Berkowitz and LePage study suggests that aggression is most likely to occur when aggressive cues are present, such as a hostile crowd or a rival player. The Daniels and Thornton study provides some evidence that aggression can be reduced in a controlled way through participation in the martial arts.

SPORT
Motivation and self-confidence in sport

STUDY 114
Gill, D. L., Dzewaltowski, D. A., 1988, 'Competitive orientations among intercollegiate athletes: is winning the only thing?', *The Sport Psychologist*, 2, 212–22

| Aim | To measure and compare levels of sport-specific achievement motivation in male and female athletes and non-athletes. |

| Method | A questionnaire. |

| Participants | The sample comprised 213 college students, separated into athletes and non-athletes and by gender. The non-athletes included 43 males and 63 females. The athletes included 59 males and 48 females. The athletes were all high-level performers at a range of different sports, including softball, swimming, track, cross-country, baseball, gymnastics and wrestling. |

| Procedure | Three questionnaires were administered to all participants at a class or team meeting, including:
1) Gill's Sport Orientation Questionnaire (SOQ), measuring achievement motivation
2) Vealey's Competitive Orientation Inventory (COI), measuring sports confidence
3) Work and Family Orientation Questionnaire (WOFO). |

| Results | Analysis of the questionnaires showed both gender differences and athlete/non-athlete differences. The gender difference was most evident for competitiveness scores, with males scoring higher than females on competitiveness and win orientation. Athletes scored higher than non-athletes on most measures, but especially so on the sport-specific competitiveness score. Athletes also placed more emphasis on performance and less on outcome than non-athletes did. Considerable variations were found between the different sports generally, reflecting the competitive structure of the activity. |

STUDY 115

Fodero, J. M., 1976, 'An analysis of achievement motivation and motivational tendencies among men and women collegiate gymnasts', *International Journal of Sports Psychology*, 11, 100–12

Aim

To measure and compare levels of achievement motivation and motivational tendencies in male and female gymnasts at different performance levels.

Method

A questionnaire.

Participants

The initial sample comprised 73 male and 66 female volunteers from 19 nationally ranked collegiate gym teams throughout the USA. The gymnasts were classed as high-level or lower-level performers, on the basis of their mean gym scores for the season 1974–5. After withdrawing the middle 10 per cent of gymnasts, a final sample of two male and two female groups, each of 30 gymnasts, was obtained.

Procedure

Two questionnaires were administered to all participants by their team coaches:
1) the Lynn Achievement Motivation Questionnaire – an eight-item list of self-referrent statements relating to Need to Achieve (Nach) – was used to measure achievement motivation
2) motivational tendencies were assessed using the Berlin Q Sort – a 60-item list of statements which participants were required to rank from most to least like themselves.

Results

Analysis of the Lynn Achievement Motivation Questionnaire showed no significant differences between males and females or between different performance levels in achievement motivation.

Analysis of the Berlin Q Sort showed no significant differences between males and females or between different performance levels in motivational tendencies.

It was concluded that men and women gymnasts, whether high- or lower-level performers, are more alike than different regarding their need to achieve and their motivational tendencies in gymnastics competition.

STUDY 116

Lepper, M. R., Greene, D., 1975, 'Turning play into work: effects of adult surveillance and extrinsic rewards on children's intrinsic motivation', *Journal of Personality and Social Psychology*, 31, 479–86

| Aim | To examine the effects of extrinsic rewards on children's intrinsic motivation. |

Method

A field experiment.

Participants

80 pre-school children aged 4–5 years, selected from the student population at the Bing Nursery School on the Stanford University Campus.

Procedure

Under two different conditions, the children were each given a set of ten geometric jigsaw puzzles to complete. (These puzzles had been pre-tested and shown to have high interest.)

In the expected reward condition the children were also shown a set of highly attractive toys – such as dolls, a garage and cars – and asked if they would like to play with them. They were then told that they would be allowed to play with them as a reward for completing the puzzles as quickly as possible – the quicker they completed them, the longer they would have to play with the toys.

In the unexpected reward condition the children were not shown the attractive toys until after they had completed the puzzles. In this condition the experimenter also stressed that they should complete the puzzles as quickly as possible.

After completing the puzzles all children were praised and allowed to play with the toys for ten minutes.

Three weeks later all the children were given the opportunity to play with the puzzles, along with other toys, as part of a normal nursery session. Intrinsic interest in the puzzles was measured by the amount of time the children spent playing with them.

Results

The results showed that the children in the expected reward condition spent less time playing with the puzzles than those in the unexpected reward condition. Hence expectation and receipt of an extrinsic reward for engaging in an activity was sufficient to produce decreased intrinsic interest in the activity.

STUDY 117

Lerner, B. S., Locke, E. A., 1995, 'The effects of goal-setting, self-efficacy, competition and personal traits on the performance of an endurance task', *Journal of Sport and Exercise Psychology*, 17, 138–52

Aim	To investigate the effects of goal-setting, self-efficacy, competition and personality on the performance of a sit-up task.
Method	A laboratory experiment.
Participants	75 male PE students (mean age = 20.4 years), who volunteered in order to gain course credits.
Procedure	Participants were randomly assigned to one of five conditions: 1) competition with hard goal 2) competition with medium goal 3) no competition with hard goal 4) no competition with medium goal 5) do best control condition. The task involved a one-minute sit-up endurance test, performed three times, with a seven-minute rest between each trial. Participants in the competition groups performed the task against a confederate, with the confederate performing first and the participant instructed to try to match or exceed their performance. Participants in the non-competition groups performed the task alone and were instructed to try to attain or exceed the assigned goals. The targets for the hard goal groups were to perform 52 sit-ups in the first trial, 51 in the second trial and 48 in the third trial. The targets for the medium goal groups were to perform 44 sit-ups in the first trial, 43 in the second trial and 38 in the third trial. Participants in the do best condition performed the task alone and were told to try their best in all trials. They were given a verbal task to complete while they performed in order to prevent them from counting their scores. Before completing the test all participants completed the Sport Orientation Questionnaire, measuring achievement motivation. Before each trial participants completed a questionnaire measuring goal commitment and provided measures of their self-efficacy by indicating how confident they were of achieving success in their next trial, on a scale of 1–10.
Results	Medium and hard goal groups significantly outperformed the do best group. Competition did not affect performance, personal goals, commitment or self-efficacy. There was a significant positive correlation between achievement motivation and performance.

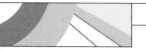

STUDY GUIDE for OCR Psychology: A2 Level

Evaluating research into motivation and self-confidence in sport

Sampling

The sample used in the Lerner and Locke study was made up of male students. This could be considered a biased sample as students are typically different to the rest of the population in many ways (e.g. they may be more used to competition and setting personal goals). They also volunteered in order to gain course credits, which is likely to make them more cooperative and helpful than the rest of the population. The sample in the Lepper and Greene study comprised children aged 4–5 years. The problem with this sample is that they are of a specific age group, which makes generalization to other age groups difficult. They are also from the same nursery school and particular features of this nursery may have contributed to the behaviour of the children (e.g. if the carers frequently used rewards as a way of encouraging the children).

Reinforcement

A reinforcer is something that increases the likelihood of a behaviour reoccurring. Reinforcers can be used to encourage or improve behaviour or performance. In the Lerner and Locke study an explanation for the superior performance of the goal-setting groups could be that they received reinforcement in the form of achieving their goal. The do best group had no such reinforcement. However, in the Lepper and Greene study they found that the expectation and receipt of reinforcement in the form of extrinsic rewards reduced intrinsic interest in the activity.

Data

One of the most common methods of measuring motivation and self-confidence is through questionnaires. A range of questionnaires was used in the studies described, all of which produce quantitative data. Such numerical data have the advantage of being easily compared and statistically analysed. However, what they do not provide is any qualitative, or descriptive, data. For example, the study by Lerner and Locke tells us that the goal-setting groups outperformed the do best group, but does not provide any descriptions of their performance. Similarly, the Gill and Dzewaltowski study tells us that males score higher than females on competitiveness and win orientation, but does not provide any data which could explain this gender difference. The focus on quantitative data in these studies leads to the problem of reductionism, where the complex psychological phenomena of motivation and self-confidence are reduced to a much simpler level, focusing on a single factor (i.e. a score on a questionnaire).

Usefulness/practical applications

Motivation and self-confidence are very important aspects of sports performance. Hence, any research that tells us more about how to improve motivation and increase self-confidence is likely to be useful to both sports performers and sports coaches. The Gill and Dzewaltowski study tells us about differences in motivation and self-confidence between males and females and between athletes and non-athletes. However, the Fodero study contradicts this to some extent, concluding that male and female gymnasts of differing performance levels are more alike than different in terms of motivation. The Lerner and Locke study suggests goal-setting as a strategy for improving motivation and performance. The Lepper and Greene study warns us of the dangers of the overuse of extrinsic rewards, particularly with children.

SPORT
Arousal and anxiety in sport

STUDY 118
Burton, D., 1988, 'Do anxious swimmers swim slower? Re-examining the elusive anxiety–performance relationship', *Journal of Sport and Exercise Psychology*, 10, 105–32

Aim

To examine the relationship between anxiety and performance in competitive swimmers, using a multidimensional approach.

Method

A correlational study, with the following hypotheses:
1) cognitive anxiety will be more consistently and strongly related to performance than somatic anxiety
2) somatic anxiety will demonstrate an inverted-U relationship with performance, whereas self-confidence and performance will exhibit a positive linear relationship and cognitive anxiety and performance will exhibit a negative one
3) short duration and high and low complexity events will demonstrate stronger relationships between somatic anxiety and performance than will long duration or moderate complexity events.

Participants

In order to test all hypotheses, two separate samples were required:
1) 15 male and 13 female collegiate swimmers (aged 18–23 years)
2) 31 male and 39 female collegiate swimmers (mean age = 17.4 years).
All swimmers were volunteers and informed consent was gained.

Procedure

All participants completed the CSAI-2, which measures cognitive state anxiety, somatic state anxiety and self-confidence.

Sample 1 completed the CSAI-2 three times during the swimming season – early, mid- and late season. Sample 2 completed the CSAI-2 twice, first following a practice session, two days prior to competition, and then one hour prior to the swimmer's most important race of the competition. Performance was measured by comparing a swimmer's performance in each race with their previous personal best and subtracting that personal best from their time in this competition. These figures were then adjusted so that comparisons could be made between races of different distances.

Results

Correlational analysis of results confirmed all three hypotheses. The general conclusions reached were that cognitive anxiety has a more damaging effect on performance than somatic anxiety; the three dimensions of anxiety have different effects on performance; somatic anxiety is more damaging to short duration and high and low complexity events than long duration or moderate complexity events; and anxious swimmers do swim slower.

STUDY 119
Bird, A. M., Horn, M. A., 1990, 'Cognitive anxiety and mental errors in sport', *Journal of Sport and Exercise Psychology*, 12, 211–16

| Aim | To test the relationship between cognitive anxiety and degree of mental errors in a sports setting. |

Aim
To test the relationship between cognitive anxiety and degree of mental errors in a sports setting.

Method
A field experiment.

Participants
Initial sample of 202 female league softball players, aged 14–17 years. Final sample of 161 participants, including 118 low in mental errors and 43 high in mental errors. Informed consent was gained from participants and teachers/coaches.

Procedure
The CSAI-2, measuring cognitive anxiety, somatic anxiety and self-confidence, was administered to the participants approximately one hour before a softball game. Measures were then taken of mental errors occurring during the game, using a Mental Errors Questionnaire designed by the researchers and completed by the coach as he observed the game. The questionnaire measured the degree to which each player's performance was adversely affected during the game compared with her usual performance during practice, using a 10-point rating scale, ranging from 'very much affected' to 'very little affected'. Analysis of these questionnaires enabled the two final groups of participants to be identified – those high in mental errors and those low in mental errors. The CSAI-2 questionnaires were then analysed in order to identify differences in anxiety between the high mental errors group and the low mental errors group. Hence the IV was high or low mental errors and the DV was anxiety score on CSAI-2.

Results
The high mental errors group had significantly higher levels of cognitive anxiety than the low mental errors group. No significant differences were found between the two groups in somatic anxiety or self-confidence. The conclusion reached was that elevations in cognitive anxiety are directly related to increases in mental errors in sports performance.

> ### STUDY 120
> Weinberg, R. S., Hunt, U. V., 1976, 'The relationship between anxiety, motor performance and electromyography', *Journal of Motor Behaviour*, 8, 219–24

| Aim | To examine the effects of anxiety on muscle tension, coordination and performance during the completion of a sports skill under stressful cconditions. |

| Method | A laboratory experiment. |

| Participants | A sample of 175 male students at the University of California. The State–Trait Anxiety Inventory (STAI) was administered to all participants and a sample of ten high-anxiety (upper 80 per cent) and ten low-anxiety (lower 20 per cent) participants was selected. Hence the final sample comprised 20. |

| Procedure | Electrodes were placed on the upper and lower arm of all participants to measure muscular activity. Participants completed an A-State questionnaire measuring state anxiety. They then completed ten trials involving throwing tennis balls at a target; the accuracy of their throws was measured and recorded. Participants were given negative feedback regarding how their performance compared with other college students. Participants completed a further ten trials. |

| Results | More anxiety was created in high-anxiety participants compared to low-anxiety participants. Performance scores showed that low-anxiety participants achieved significantly higher scores than high-anxiety participants after failure feedback.

The electromyographic recordings indicated that high-anxiety participants used more energy before, during and after the throws than did low-anxiety participants. |

Evaluating research into arousal and anxiety in sport

Methods of measurement

The three most common methods of measuring arousal and anxiety are questionnaires, physiological measures and observation. Questionnaires include the Competitive State Anxiety Inventory (CSAI) and the Sports Competition Anxiety Test (SCAT). Physiological measures involve measuring changes in physiological indicators of arousal, such as heart rate, muscle tension and breathing rate. Observational methods involve observing and recording behavioural indicators of anxiety, such as biting nails, fiddling with clothes or touching face, as well as changes in performance. These methods all have strengths and weaknesses. The questionnaire method used in the studies by Burton and Bird and Horn is probably the easiest, as large amounts of data can be gathered quickly and the method can be used in a sports setting. However, questionnaires are subject to bias in that participants may respond to demand characteristics or be influenced by social desirability. Participants may also have difficulty understanding the questions or applying the descriptions to themselves. Limited response options may also make selecting answers difficult. The Weinberg and Hunt study used both physiological

231

and observational methods. The advantages of physiological methods are that they are scientific and reliable and are not open to bias. However, they are impractical in a sports setting. Observational methods can easily be used in a sports setting, but they are subject to observer bias and results are often difficult to analyse.

Data
Both the questionnaire method used in the Burton and Bird and Horn studies and the physiological method used in the Weinberg and Hunt study produced quantitative data, which can be analysed easily and allows comparisons to be made. However, qualitative descriptions and explanations are lacking and it could be argued that these studies provide a reductionist view of anxiety.

Usefulness/practical applications
These studies show that for many athletes performance deteriorates when they are anxious and that cognitive anxiety is the most damaging. Research into anxiety and sports performance, which tells us more about when and how anxiety is likely to affect performance, is useful to athletes and coaches, who can use this information to try to develop strategies to control or reduce anxiety, thereby minimizing its effects on performance. According to the results of Burton and Bird and Horn, these strategies should focus on cognitive anxiety.

SPORT
Attitudes to exercise and sport

STUDY 121
Garcia, A. W., King, A. C., 1991, 'Predicting long-term adherence to aerobic exercise', *Journal of Sport and Exercise Psychology*, 13, 394–410

| Aim | To identify the factors that contribute to long-term participation in aerobic exercise. |

Aim To identify the factors that contribute to long-term participation in aerobic exercise.

Method A field experiment.

Participants 74 sedentary, healthy men and women (42 male, 32 female), aged 50–64 years, who responded to advertisements in north California. The majority were white and well educated (three years at college) and two-thirds were married.

Procedure Participants were randomly assigned to one of four conditions:
1) 'assessment-only' control, where participants were asked not to change their activity habits over the following 12 months
2) 'moderate-intensity group' condition, where participants were asked to attend three one-hour exercise classes per week where they exercised at 65–80 per cent of their maximum capacity
3) 'moderate-intensity home-based' condition, where participants were provided with an exercise programme identical in terms of frequency, duration and intensity to the one used in the moderate-intensity group condition
4) 'low-intensity home-based' condition, where the same general instructions and approach were used as for the moderate-intensity home-based condition, except that participants exercised at 50–60 per cent of their maximum capacity and were instructed to exercise for five 30-minute sessions per week.

Following completion of each class, participants completed an attendance log recording information concerning that day's exercise session, including perceived exertion, enjoyment and convenience (PEEC) as well as the duration of the exercise and maximal heart rate achieved. At the start, at six months and at one year participants completed a battery of physiological and psychological tests including a self-motivation inventory and a self-efficacy scale.

Results Perceived exertion, enjoyment and convenience were not found to be significantly related to exercise adherence. Similarly, self-motivation was not significantly related to adherence. Results showed that self-efficacy was strongly related to exercise adherence, however. These results suggest that self-efficacy, conceptualised as one's belief at a particular point in time that one can perform a specific behaviour, is the most important factor in encouraging continued participation in exercise.

STUDY 122
Gill, D. L., Gross, J. B., Huddleston, S., 1979, 'Participation motivation in youth sports', *International Journal of Sports Psychology*, 14, 1–14

| Aim | To identify reasons for participation in youth sports. |

Method

A questionnaire.

Participants

1138 youths (720 boys, 418 girls), aged 8–18 years, attending Iowa Summer Sports School, participating in a wide range of sports.

Procedure

A questionnaire consisting of a list of 30 possible reasons for participating in sport (see table below) was administered to all participants at three sessions, each lasting one week, during June–July 1979. The questionnaire asked participants to rate each reason on a three-point scale ('important', 'somewhat important', 'not at all important').

Results

Combined gender analysis showed 'improving skills' to have the highest rating, followed by 'fun', 'learn new skills', 'challenge' and 'fitness'. Separate gender analysis showed that both boys and girls rated 'improving skills' the highest, but girls then rated 'fun' as second, whereas boys rated 'challenge' as second.

Reasons	Mean ratings		
	Boys	Girls	Combined
I want to improve my skills	1.06	1.09	1.07
I want to be with my friends	2.00	2.00	2.00
I like to win	1.40	1.93	1.59
I want to get rid of energy	2.55	2.41	2.50
I like to travel	2.33	2.34	2.33
I want to stay in shape	1.36	1.30	1.34
I like the excitement	1.37	1.30	1.34
I like the teamwork	1.42	1.30	1.38
My parents or close friends want me to play	2.27	2.53	2.36
I want to learn new skills	1.18	1.13	1.16
I like to meet new friends	1.59	1.38	1.51
I like to do something I'm good at	1.31	1.47	1.37
I want to release tension	2.27	2.36	2.31
I like the rewards	2.62	1.96	1.75
I like to get exercise	1.46	1.28	1.39
I like to have something to do	1.81	1.69	1.77
I like the action	1.32	1.31	1.32
I like the team spirit	1.40	1.31	1.37
I like to get out of the house	2.10	2.21	2.14
I like to compete	1.17	1.15	1.30
I like to feel important	1.67	1.90	1.75
I like being on a team	1.39	1.22	1.39
I want to go on to a higher level	1.23	1.45	1.31
I want to be physically fit	1.24	1.40	1.23
I want to be popular	2.02	2.47	2.18
I like the challenge	1.16	1.28	1.20
I like the coaches or instructors	1.71	1.76	1.73
I want to gain status or recognition	1.72	2.16	1.88
I like to have fun	1.17	1.11	1.15
I like to use the equipment or facilities	1.83	1.89	1.85

STUDY 123
Stevens, M. J., Lane, A. M., 2001, 'Mood-regulating strategies used by athletes', *Athletic Insight*, 13, 3

| Aim | To investigate the strategies used by athletes to regulate moods. |

Aim To investigate the strategies used by athletes to regulate moods.

Method A questionnaire.

Participants 107 athletes (64 male, 43 female, mean age = 19.6 years) from undergraduate sports science courses at universities in the UK. All participants were at least county standard in one of the following sports: badminton, basketball, hockey, karate, netball, rugby, football, swimming, track and field.

Procedure The Self-Regulating Strategies of Mood Questionnaire was administered to all participants away from the site of competition. The questionnaire listed 29 strategies thought to influence moods – for example, listening to music, going shopping, exercising, talking to someone. Participants were asked to nominate strategies they used to change specific moods and to rate the effectiveness of each strategy (on a nine-point scale, from 'not at all effective' to 'extremely effective'). The moods stated were those measured by the Profile of Mood States questionnaire, including anger, confusion, depression, fatigue, tension and vigour.

Results Exercise was one of only three strategies identified as being used to regulate all six moods, the others being 'listen to music' and 'change location'. There were strategies unique to certain mood dimensions: 'try to be alone' for anger; 'analyse the situation' for confusion; 'engage in pleasant activities' for depression; and 'use relaxation techniques' for tension. The findings support the notion that mood can be controlled by the individual and that exercise is associated with improved mood. However, the mechanisms that bring about improved mood are unclear.

STUDY 124

Morgan, W. P., Brown, D. R., Raglin, J. S., O'Connor, P. J., Ellickson, K. A., 1987, 'Psychological monitoring of overtraining and staleness', *British Journal of Sports Medicine*, 21, 107–14

| Aim | To investigate the effects of training on mood states. |

| Method | A longitudinal questionnaire study. |

| Participants | Approximately 200 men and 200 women members of the University of Wisconsin-Madison swimming teams during the period 1975–86. |

| Procedure | Participants completed the Profile of Mood States (POMS) questionnaire at regular intervals (ranging from two to four weeks) during one swimming season in the period 1975–86. The questionnaire measures the mood that is temporarily created by being in a particular situation, measuring the following mood states:
1) tension
2) depression
3) anger
4) vigour
5) fatigue
6) confusion. |

| Results | The results indicate that mood state disturbances increased as the training increased and that these mood disturbances fell to baseline levels with reduction of the training load. These results suggest that monitoring of mood states provides a potential method of preventing staleness. |

Evaluating research into attitudes to exercise and sport

Sampling

The study by Stevens and Lane used students as the participants and it can be argued that there are differences between students and non-students which may be relevant to the research question in this study, e.g. their social habits, and may influence the results. Hence results from samples of students are not easily generalizable to the rest of the population. In contrast, the sample used in the Garcia and King study comprised men and women aged 50–64 years. This is interesting as this advanced age group are not often studied in sports research. However, the sample is biased by the fact that the majority were white, well educated and married. The Gill *et al.* study provides a very large sample of young people of a fairly wide age range, participating in a wide range of sports.

Questionnaires

Questionnaires feature strongly in research into attitudes to exercise and sport. In the Gill *et al.* study they were used to identify reasons for participation in sport; in the Garcia and King study self-motivation and self-efficacy were measured; Stevens and Lane used questionnaires to identify strategies to change moods; and Morgan *et al.* used the POMS questionnaire to measure mood states.

Questionnaires are a convenient method of collecting data; they are quick and easy to administer and large sets of data can be gained. However, questionnaires also have limitations: situational factors may influence participants' responses; closed questions or limited response options often provide a restricted picture; and participants may be influenced by demand characteristics or demonstrate a social desirability bias. These limitations may reduce the reliability and validity of the results.

The POMS questionnaire used in the Morgan *et al.* study and referred to in the Stevens and Lane study was originally developed for use in the clinical field and, despite adaptations made to utilize it in the sports arena, it has been argued that the sense of measuring psychological disturbance still remains, hence reducing its effectiveness.

Usefulness/practical applications

Research into attitudes to exercise and sport is useful as it helps us to understand why people participate in sport and how to encourage those who do not. This is obviously valuable information that has wider implications for today's society, with children spending more and more time sitting in front of television and computer screens and with obesity and heart disease on the increase, constituting a major drain on NHS resources. The Gill *et al.* and Garcia and King studies give us an insight into how to encourage both young and elderly people to become involved in sport; the Stevens and Lane study tells us of the benefits of exercise for improving mood states; however, the Morgan *et al.* study warns us of the dangers of excessive exercise.

STUDY 125
Sherif, M., 1956, 'Experiments in group conflict', *Scientific American*, 195, 54–8

Aim	To study informal groups and observe the natural development of group organization and attitudes. To see if competition will create hostility.

Method	A field experiment.

Participants	Boys aged 11–12 years, selected by a long and thorough procedure involving interviews with family, teachers and school officials, and also school and medical records, personality tests and observations in class and at play. The boys were unknown to each other and were all healthy, socially well adjusted, above-average intelligence and from stable, white, Protestant, middle-class homes. The sample was deliberately homogeneous to reduce the chances of bringing established social conflicts to the study. The participants were unaware that they were part of an experiment.

Procedure
The experimenters created an isolated summer camp which the boys attended. The researchers played the role of camp leaders. The study included three phases:
1) The boys were all housed together in a large bunk house and the experimenters observed the development of group structure; after a few days they divided the boys into two groups, deliberately separating 'best friends', and gave them a range of challenging activities, e.g. hikes, sports, camp-outs, to complete.
2) Conflict was introduced through competition, with the groups competing against each other in various games, which resulted in increasing hostility between the groups.
3) The researchers reconciled the two groups by creating common tasks for them to complete, creating a series of urgent and natural situations, e.g. making the camp truck break down, which had to be resolved by the boys pulling the truck together.

Results
The study produced the following results for each phase:
1) Clear social hierarchies developed in both groups with leaders and lieutenants emerging who were rated more positively by the other boys.
2) They began calling each other names, turning against previous friends, refusing contact with members of the other group and rating boys in the other group very negatively; solidarity increased within each group.
3) The hostility between the groups quickly broke down and the boys developed new friendships with members of the other group.

This study shows how social hierarchies naturally develop in groups. It also shows how easily competition can lead to conflict between groups. Finally it shows how common goals can break down the barriers and reduce hostility between competing groups.

STUDY 126
Slater, M. R., Sewell, D. F., 1994, 'An examination of the cohesion–performance relationship in university hockey teams', *Journal of Sports Sciences*, 12, 423–31

| Aim | To assess whether team cohesion in university-level field hockey was a cause for, or an effect of, successful performance. |

Aim   To assess whether team cohesion in university-level field hockey was a cause for, or an effect of, successful performance.

Method   Correlation.

Participants   60 hockey players, aged 18–24 years, competing at university level at the University of Hull, including three men's teams (n = 29) and three women's teams (n = 31).

Procedure   Team cohesion was measured using the Group Environment Questionnaire (GEQ), which assesses task and social cohesion. The questionnaire comprises 18 items, each rated on a nine-point scale, ranging from 'strongly agree' to 'strongly disagree'. The four aspects assessed by the questionnaire were:
1) attraction to social aspects of the group
2) attraction to group's task
3) perception of group's social integration
4) perception of group's integration around its task.
The questionnaires were completed twice by each participant, once midway through the season and then again four weeks later. Scores on this questionnaire were correlated with team performance, measured by the number of points achieved in the previous five games, with 2 points given for a win, 1 point for a draw and 0 points for a loss. Participants were made aware of the purpose of the study after the questionnaires had been completed for the second time.

Results   Positive correlations were found between team cohesion and performance outcome, i.e. higher team cohesiveness, more successful performance. Social cohesion was more highly associated with performance than task cohesion. Cohesion had more influence on performance than performance did on cohesion.

STUDY 127
Schwartz, B., Barsky, S. F., 1977, 'The home advantage', *Social Forces*, 55, 641–61

Aim	To investigate the existence of the home advantage in ice hockey, basketball, baseball and football.
Method	Indirect observation.
Participants	Details of the following sports events: 1) major league baseball matches in 1971 2) US football games in 1971 3) national ice hockey league matches in 1971 4) collegiate basketball matches over 15 years (1952–66).
Procedure	Data were analysed for each sport on the following: location of games, outcome of games, team's standing at time of game and attendance figures. Home advantage was measured by the degree to which home victories exceeded 50 per cent of the games won.
Results	A home advantage was seen in all sports, but the extent of that advantage differed from one sport to another. The percentage of home wins for each sport were as follows: 1) baseball 53 per cent 2) football 60 per cent 3) ice hockey 64 per cent 4) basketball 64 per cent. The authors considered three possible explanations for the home advantage, including:

Familiarity with the home arena and playing area – this was discounted as an explanation as the greatest home advantage was seen in the sports with the most uniform playing areas, which are least affected by environmental variations.

Travel fatigue in the away team – this was discounted as an explanation by the authors as they felt that the home advantage should increase as the season progresses due to the effects of injuries and wear and tear becoming more aggravated by travel if this explanation were correct. However, they found no significant tendency for the home advantage to increase as the season progressed.

Moral support from home spectators – the authors concluded that the home advantage was primarily due to the moral support given by home spectators. They suggested that the home team were motivated to try harder in order to gain the reward of social approval.

Evaluating research into social influence in sport

Ecological validity
All three studies could be considered to have high ecological validity as they all involve studying participants in a fairly natural environment. The Sherif study took

place in a children's summer camp and the participants were unaware that they were part of an experiment. In the Slater and Sewell study participants were studied during the course of a hockey season. The Schwartz and Barsky study involved indirect observation of various sports events conducted some time after the events had taken place. None of these studies involved obvious manipulation or control of participants, which makes it easier to generalize the results to everyday situations.

Ethics

Research into social psychology can suffer with ethical problems. In the Sherif study the researchers did gain parental consent but deceived the boys, in that they were unaware that they were part of an experiment and were being observed. It could also be argued that the researchers encouraged, or at least provided the opportunity for, the boys to develop and demonstrate hostility towards each other. The boys showed ethnocentrism, or the tendency to favour their own group and see it as superior to others. This is the basis for prejudice and discrimination. In the Slater and Sewell study the participants were not informed of the purpose of the study until the end and so could not give fully informed consent. In the Schwartz and Barsky study it is unlikely that permission was gained from the participants in the sports events studied.

Data

In both the Schwartz and Barsky and Slater and Sewell studies quantitative data were gained through questionnaires or analysis of events. The data in the Schwartz and Barsky study were extensive as they included details of a number of different sports events over an extended period of time. This numerical data allowed for comparisons between different sports in terms of home advantage. The quantitative data in the Slater and Sewell study included questionnaire scores and performance measurements and allowed for correlational analysis to establish the relationship between group cohesion and performance. In the Sherif study data were collected through observations, providing qualitative data. Such data are generally rich in detail and can provide both descriptions and possible explanations for behaviour. However, qualitative data are typically difficult to analyse.

Usefulness/practical applications

Most sports take place in a social setting and so research into social behaviour is likely to be relevant. Research can tell us how the presence of others is likely to influence our behaviour and affect our sports performance. The Sherif study tells us what may happen when groups are competing against each other and suggests a way of reducing conflict and hostility between groups. This has relevance for anyone involved in team sports, particularly those involving young children. The Slater and Sewell study shows us how important group cohesion is for successful team performance, suggesting that coaches should focus on developing strategies to increase group cohesion in order to improve performance. The study by Schwartz and Barsky provides evidence of the home advantage in a number of sports and gives an explanation for this advantage. This could lead to coaches developing strategies to maximize the home advantage (and minimize the away disadvantage) for their teams.

STUDY 128

Lewin, K., Lippit, R., White, R. K., 1939, 'Patterns of aggressive behaviour in experimentally created social climates', *Journal of Social Psychology*, 10, 271–99

Aim

To study behavioural responses to different leadership styles, including authoritarian, democratic and *laissez-faire*.

Method

A field experiment.

Participants

A sample of 20 boys, aged ten years, divided into four groups of five, with each group pre-matched in terms of physical, intellectual and social ability. Parental consent was gained.

Procedure

The experiment took place over a period of five months during which the boys attended a children's activity club. Each group had a leader who used one of the following leadership styles:

Authoritarian – where the leader dictates to the group *who* does *what* and *how*, and advice, ideas or comments are not asked for.

Democratic – where the leader encourages the involvement of the members of the group, their ideas are listened to and they are encouraged to participate in decisions relating to the execution of group tasks.

Laissez-faire – where leaders offer no direction and group members are left to get on with things in their own way.

Every six weeks each group had a new leader using a new leadership style. All leaders used each style and all groups had each leader using each style.

Data were collected using observation, video and audio recordings and interviews with children, parents, teachers and leaders. Social interactions within the groups were analysed, with particular emphasis on aggressive behaviour.

Results

With the authoritarian-style leader the groups were most productive, but tended to stop or slow down their work when the leader was absent and became aggressive towards each other when things went wrong. With the democratic leader the groups were slightly less productive, but continued to work on their tasks when the leader was absent and cooperated when things went wrong. With the *laissez-faire*-style leader members were least productive and tended to be aggressive towards each other and gave up easily when things went wrong.

STUDY 129
Carron, A. V., Bennet, B. B., 1977, 'Compatibility in the coach–athlete dyad', *Research Quarterly*, 48, 671–9

Aim

To examine the factors contributing to effective interpersonal interaction between coaches and athletes.

Method

An experiment using questionnaires.

Participants

54 coach–athlete dyads (36 compatible, 18 incompatible) comprising college coaches and male and female student athletes from a range of sports. Compatible and incompatible athletes were identified by the coaches.

Procedure

The Fundamental Interpersonal Relations Orientation-Behaviour (FIRO-B) questionnaire was administered to both coaches and athletes. It assessed:
1) inclusion – levels of communication and interaction
2) control – authority, power and dominance
3) affection – close personal feeling.
The questionnaire measured behaviour towards others and desired behaviour towards self.
   The hypothesis predicted that the biggest differences between the compatible and incompatible dyads would be in the areas of affection and control.

Results

Differences were found in the areas of affection and control, but contrary to the hypothesis the biggest differences were in inclusion i.e. levels of communication and interaction between coaches and athletes.

STUDY 130
Barnett, N. P., Smoll, F. L., Smith, R. E., 1992, 'Effects of enhancing coach–athlete relationships on youth sport attrition', *The Sport Psychologist*, 6, 111–27

Aim

To examine the impact of the Coach Effectiveness Training Programme on children's attitudes towards participation in baseball.

Method

A field experiment.

Participants

18 male baseball coaches and 202 baseball players aged 10–11 years.

Procedure

Eight coaches attended a pre-season Coach Effectiveness Training programme designed to facilitate desirable coach–athlete interactions. These formed the experimental group. The remaining ten coaches did not attend any pre-season courses and formed the control group. Each coach was responsible for a baseball team for a season.

Data were collected from the children through interviews and questionnaires completed before the season started, after the season finished and before the following season began. Information included evaluations of the coach, team-mates and baseball itself.

Anonymity was assured, with each child given a code number and no names recorded.

Results

Experimental groups evaluated coach, team-mates and baseball more positively than the control groups. Player attrition for the following season was higher for the control group (26 per cent) than for the experimental group (5 per cent).

Evaluating research into leadership and coaching

Research methods
The research method used in both the Lewin *et al.* and Barnett *et al.* studies was field experiment. Here the researcher has less control over variables than with laboratory experiments, but gains in terms of ecological validity. In the Lewin *et al.* study the participants were attending a children's activity club over a period of five months. This would be a fairly normal environment for children and not one that has been created by the researchers for the purposes of the experiment. In the Barnett *et al.* study the participants were members of a baseball team and were studied throughout the course of one season – again, a natural environment. The advantage of studying people in their natural environment is that they are more likely to display natural behaviour and it makes generalizations to real-life situations easier.

Sampling

The sample in the Lewin *et al.* study comprised 20 boys, aged ten years, divided into four groups of five. A sample of five is very small and would have the disadvantage that individual differences between participants may influence the results e.g. if one boy was particularly aggressive. However, in this study, the researchers pre-matched the groups, making them as similar as possible, which would reduce the effects of any individual differences.

In the Carron and Bennet study the sample comprised college coaches and student athletes. The fact that they were all in an educational environment may make their relationships different to coach–athlete relationships in other settings e.g. the students may be dependent upon the coaches for educational assessments. The compatible and incompatible pairs were identified by the coaches, which is subjective and open to bias. The student (or an independent observer) may have a different view of the relationship.

The sample in the Barnett *et al.* study included 18 male coaches. The number of coaches in the experimental group was just eight, which again creates the possibility of individual differences influencing results. It is possible that a number of these coaches were simply better coaches to start with.

Data

Data were collected in the Carron and Bennet study by means of questionnaires. This provided quantitative data, which have the advantage of being easily analysed. However, it provides no qualitative descriptions or explanations of behaviour e.g. it does not tell us anything about the communication and interaction between the coaches and athletes. The Barnett *et al.* and Lewin *et al.* studies both provide qualitative data from interviews or observations, which are far richer in detail but often have the disadvantage of being difficult to analyse.

Use of interviews

Two of the studies described use interviews as one of the methods of collecting data. As both these studies include fairly young children it is worth noting that demand characteristics may influence them and they may display a social desirability bias, particularly as they may have been questioned about their adult leaders. Children of this age may find it difficult to voice any negative views about adults.

SPORT
Attention and imagery in sport

STUDY 131
Baghurst, T., Thierry, G., Holder, T., 2003, 'Evidence for a relationship between attentional style and effective cognitive strategies during performance', *Athletic Insight*, 6

Aim

To determine a relationship between attentional styles and attentional strategies during sports performance.

Method

A laboratory experiment.

Participants

60 Bangor University Sports Science students, mean age 22.5 years. All were novice rowers but were familiar with the technique. The sample was reduced to 14 (two female, 12 male) through a Test of Attentional and Interpersonal Style (TAIS) selection process which identified seven as internalizers and seven as externalizers.

Procedure

All participants completed an informed consent form and health questionnaire and were assured of confidentiality. All participants completed the TAIS, which identifies attentional style. This was analysed to identify clear 'internalizers' (those who tend to focus their attention internally) and 'externalizers' (those who tend to focus their attention externally).

Using a counterbalanced design, each participant completed two 15-minute maximum rowing exercises, each time using a different attentional strategy during performance. One was in an 'associative' condition where they were instructed to focus their attention on a digital display showing details of their current performance (such as distance completed, 500 split, stroke rate per minute and a countdown of time). They were requested to read aloud total distance covered every 15 seconds to ensure that they were focusing on the display, and therefore associating. The second performance was in a 'dissociative' condition where they were unable to see the digital display and were asked to answer simple flash card multiplication questions, thereby preventing them from focusing their performance and forcing them to dissociate.

Participants completed a post-exercise questionnaire evaluating their performance at the end of each trial in terms of how easy they found it to adhere to the attentional strategy assigned, how difficult they found it to concentrate on the task and which strategies they would use in future.

Results

The associative condition produced better performance in internalizers. The dissociative condition produced better performance in externalizers. Participants found it significantly more difficult to adhere to their 'non-preferred' attentional strategy, clearly favouring the strategy most similar to their attentional style. The majority indicated that they would employ this attentional strategy in future.

STUDY 132
Slade, J. M., Landers, D. M., Martin, P. E., 2002, 'Muscular activity during real and imagined movements', *Journal of Sport and Exercise Psychology*, 24, 151–67

| Aim | To examine whether muscular activity occurs during an imagined dumb-bell curl. To see whether the activity mirrors that which occurs during the actual performance of the skill. To see whether muscular activity is greater in participants who are aware of the prediction than those who are unaware. |

Aim

To examine whether muscular activity occurs during an imagined dumb-bell curl. To see whether the activity mirrors that which occurs during the actual performance of the skill. To see whether muscular activity is greater in participants who are aware of the prediction than those who are unaware.

Method

A laboratory experiment.

Participants

60 Arizona State University students (38 male, 22 female), aged 19–36 years, divided into two groups of 30 – 'theory aware' and 'theory unaware'.

Procedure

1) EMG electrodes were attached to participants' arms and baseline measures of muscular activity were recorded at rest
2) the 'theory aware' group was informed of the hypothesis regarding muscular activity during imagery; the 'theory unaware' group was not informed
3) each participant performed six dumb-bell curls with EMG activity measured
4) participants relaxed for one minute
5) each participant imagined performing six dumb-bell curls; EMG activity measured.

Results

EMG activity was significantly greater during imagery than at rest. EMG activity during imagery did not mirror that which occurred during actual performance. No EMG differences were found between the 'theory aware' and 'theory unaware' groups.

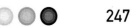

STUDY 133
Isaac, A., 1991, 'Mental practice. Does it work in the field?', *The Sports Psychologist*, 6, 192–8

Aim

To examine the effectiveness of visual mental practice on the learning of a complex physical skill in a sports setting. The influence of imagery ability was also examined.

Method

A field experiment.

Participants

78 PE students, half of whom were experienced trampolinists and half of whom were novices. All were tested for imagery ability using imagery questionnaires and were classified as either high or low imagers. The sample was divided into a control group (n = 39) and an experimental group (n = 39). Each group included both experienced and novice trampolinists and both high and low imagers.

Procedure

Both groups attempted to learn or improve three trampolining skills over three training periods of six weeks. The experimental and control groups were treated identically during training, except for the mental task during the five-minute break that occurred in each session.

At each session each group physically practised the skill for $2\frac{1}{2}$ minutes, followed by a five-minute break, during which the experimental group mentally practised the skill while the control group practised an abstract mental task e.g. mental arithmetic. Both groups then completed a further physical practice of $2\frac{1}{2}$ minutes.

Participants were videotaped performing the first and final attempt at each skill, which was then independently marked by qualified judges.

Results

Analysis of results demonstrated that the experimental group showed significantly more improvement than the control group. High imagers showed significantly more improvement than low imagers. The experts benefitted from using the imagery significantly more than the novices.

Evaluating research into attention and imagery in sport

Research methods
All three studies described use experimental methods. Slade *et al.* and Baghurst *et al.* conducted laboratory experiments. This method has the advantage of the researcher having high control over variables in the experimental setting e.g. instructions, times, trials etc. This control allows for cause-and-effect relationships to be established and makes replication possible. However, this high control is at the expense of ecological validity. Both these studies are low in ecological validity as they do not take place in an everyday environment or involve the performance of everyday tasks. The participants would have been aware that this was an experiment and may have responded to demand characteristics where they change their behaviour in some way, usually so as to cooperate with the experimenter. The study by Isaac was a field experiment, which has higher ecological validity as it involves studying the

participants in a more natural environment. However, the researcher was still manipulating the environment and the participants would have been aware that they were being studied.

Sampling

The participants used in these studies were all students. Students are often thought not to be typical of the general population and so it may be difficult to generalize the results of these studies to the rest of the population. For example, because they are in an educational environment, students may be more used to paying attention and may be better able to use and control their imagination than non-students. The sample in the Baghurst *et al.* study was also very small and individual differences between participants, for example in their ability to use the attentional strategies, may have influenced the results.

Usefulness/practical applications

These studies all show that attention and imagery can have an effect on sports performance. The Slade *et al.* study showed that muscular activity occurs during imagery and Isaac found that mental practice of a sports skill significantly improved performance. This suggests that athletes who include imagery and mental practice as part of their training schedule may have an advantage over athletes who include physical practice only. The Baghurst *et al.* research suggests that where we focus our attention during sports performance can have an impact on our level of performance. The results suggest that attentional strategies used during performance should be matched to individual attentional styles in order to maximize performance.

See also...

Studies 11, 17, 19, 20, 21, 22, 27, 33, 36, 63, 67, 68, 72, 73, 75, 76 and 135.

Section 6
CRIME

STUDY 134

Raine, A., Lui, J.-H., 1998, 'Biological predispositions to violence and their implications for biosocial treatment and prevention', *Psychology, Crime and Law*, 4, 107–25

Aim

This review article describes four recent studies conducted by the authors that identify possible biological risk factors for violence and crime (one of which is the 'murderers' brains' study that you may have looked at in the OCR AS course); two of the studies are summarized below.

Study 1 – Are low levels of physiological arousal a predictor of offending behaviour?

Method

A correlational study.

Participants

101 boys aged 15 years.

Procedure

This is a correlational study, which looked for a relationship between a number of physiological measures (skin conductance, EEG and heart rate) taken at age 15 years and the numbers of offences the participants had committed by the age of 24 years.

Results

The authors report a strong correlation between the two measures. Those committing crimes had significantly lower heart rates, reduced skin conductance and more slow-wave EEG theta activity than non-criminals. The authors claim that these measures correctly classified 74.7 per cent of all participants as criminal or non-criminal.

Study 2 – Are birth complications combined with early maternal rejection a predictor of offending behaviour?

Method

A correlational study.

Participants

4269 consecutive live male births in Copenhagen, Denmark.

Procedure

The researchers collected data on the following:
1) birth complications (including breech, forceps and anoxia)
2) maternal rejection (mother not wanting pregnancy, attempted abortion or institutionalization by four months)
3) violent crime (data collected when the participants were aged 18 years) – these crimes included murder, attempted murder, assault, rape, armed robbery, illegal possession of a firearm and threats of violence.

Results

Those boys who had experienced both birth complications and early childhood rejection were most likely to become violent offenders, although there was no effect for non-violent offending. There was also no interaction between poverty and birth complications. This is thought to be the first study to provide evidence from a large birth cohort to show that birth complications in association with rejection are associated with violent crime. The authors conclude by stating that although they have demonstrated a link between physiological functioning and criminal behaviour, it is the interaction between biological and social predisposition that is crucial to understanding violent crime.

STUDY 135

Eysenck, S. B. G., Rust, J., Eysenck, H. J., 1977, 'Personality and the classification of adult offenders', *British Journal of Criminology*, 17, 2

| Aim | An attempt to classify criminal behaviour in relation to personality variables. The personality variables measured in this study are extroversion, neuroticism and psychosis. The authors argue that these variables show strong evidence of genetic determination as well as being linked with criminal behaviour. |

Method

A correlational study.

Participants

156 prisoners, aged 18–38 years, divided into five groups on the basis of their crimes:
1) violent crimes – prisoners who had committed two or more violent crimes (no sexual crimes)
2) property crimes – prisoners with three or more convictions for breaking and entering and other convictions for theft only
3) confidence crimes (fraud) – prisoners with three or more convictions for fraud (no convictions for violent or sexual crimes)
4) inadequates – prisoners with ten or more convictions in three years and serving an average sentence of less than 18 months (no convictions for robbery and not more than one conviction for a violent or sexual offence)
5) residual – prisoners who did not fall into any of the above categories (i.e. those who committed a variety of crimes in combination).

Procedure

They were all tested on the Eysenck Personality Questionnaire (EPQ) and also on a variety of physiological measures, including skin conductance, EEG and eye blink responses.

Results

The authors claim that it is possible to classify offenders by personality types. The first major distinction was seen with the psychosis scores, with the conmen having very low scores. Neuroticism scores separated the violent and property offenders (low scores) from the inadequates and residuals (high scores). Finally, the extroversion scores distinguished between the violent and residual offenders (high scores) and the inadequates and property offenders (low scores), although this difference did not reach statistical significance.

Some physiological differences were also found between the property and inadequate offenders and the other three groups.

STUDY 136

Farrington, D. P., Barnes, G. C., Lambert, S., 1996, 'The concentration of offending in families', *Legal and Criminological Psychology*, 1, 47–63

Aim

To test the hypothesis that problem families produce problem children. The research here is part of a much larger longitudinal study, namely the Cambridge Study in Delinquent Development, which has followed a group of males from the ages of eight to 32 years in interviews and from the ages of ten to 40 years via their criminal records. This paper attempts to relate convictions of these males to the convictions of their biological parents and full biological siblings.

Method

A longitudinal study using interviews and data collected from the Criminal Records Office.

Participants

411 boys from inner-city areas of London, mostly born in 1953. Participants were selected by taking all eight- and nine-year-old boys from the registers of six state primary schools in a single location in London. The boys were predominantly white and from working-class families. As there were 14 pairs of brothers in the original sample (including five pairs of twins) there are 397 different families involved in the research. To avoid counting the same family more than once, one of each pair (the younger brother or a randomly selected twin) was excluded from this analysis.

Procedure

The Cambridge Study involved interviews with the children and their parents and questionnaires completed by the children's teachers. These results have been reported in numerous papers and books. In this study the focus was on criminal records. Searches were carried out in the central Criminal Record Office in London to locate evidence of convictions of the males, their biological fathers and mothers and their full brothers and sisters (and also their wives/partners, but these findings are not discussed here). The Criminal Record Office contains records of all relatively serious offences committed in Great Britain or Ireland and also holds records of minor juvenile offences committed in London. The records would not include details of common assault, traffic violations and drunkenness. Most commonly the offences were theft, burglary and unauthorized taking of motor vehicles, although they also included violence, vandalism, fraud and drug abuse.

Results

Earlier reports from the Cambridge Study have confirmed the hypothesis that criminals are likely to have criminal relatives. When those in the original cohort were aged 20 years, 48 per cent of those with convicted fathers also had convictions, compared to 19 per cent of those without convicted fathers. This was not dependent on when the father had committed the offence (before or after the son was born), suggesting that there was no direct behavioural influence. 54 per cent of those with convicted mothers also had convictions, compared to 23 per cent of those with mothers without convictions. This link remained even when males with both mother and father with convictions were removed from the analysis. These results are confirmed in this analysis, which took place when the study males were aged

40 years. 64 per cent of the families contained one convicted person or more, and just 6 per cent (23 families) of the families accounted for over half of all the convictions. Conviction of one family member is strongly linked to conviction of another family member. About 75 per cent of convicted parents had a convicted child, and having a sibling who had been convicted (especially an older sibling) was a strong predictor of conviction. These results are not the result of co-offending with family members. There were 26 study males who had co-offended with father, mother or sibling and when this data was excluded from the analysis the effect remained strong.

Overall, the results provide strong support for the notion that offending is concentrated in families and tends to be transmitted from one generation to the next. However, as the authors point out, these results do not establish whether this is due to the influence of nature or nurture.

Evaluating research into explanations of criminal behaviour

The nature/nurture debate
Considering the relative influence of nature and nurture in the determination of criminal behaviour is obviously crucial. We have looked at some research that considers the importance of genetic factors (Raine and Lui and Eysenck *et al.*) and some that considers the importance of environment and upbringing (Farrington *et al.*). Farrington *et al*'s research clearly suggests that environment plays a major part in criminal behaviour, and results from the Cambridge Study as a whole identify social/environmental factors – such as poverty, low family income, large family size and poor child-rearing techniques – as major influences. In the study reported here, it is clear that offending is concentrated in families and passes from generation to generation. However, this could be due to the kind of social/environmental factors mentioned above or it could be due to genetic factors. The research conducted does not allow us to discriminate between these two explanations. Raine and Lui offer strong support for the role of genetic factors in determining criminal behaviour, although they stress that it is the interaction between these factors and social environment that is crucial. Interestingly, they suggest that poverty does not contribute significantly to criminal behaviours. It is unlikely that research will ever resolve this debate. First, it is likely that criminal behaviour (as all other behaviours) is the result of a complex interaction between both nature and nurture and the vast number of different crimes makes it unlikely that a single explanation fits all. Second, it is virtually impossible to think of a piece of research that could be conducted that would answer this question. The current viewpoint would appear to be that psychology has identified a number of genetic factors (physiological, neurophysiological, personality etc.) which appear to contribute to the likelihood of someone committing a criminal offence, but that these factors are mediated by a vast array of social and environmental factors.

Correlation not causation
This is a very important evaluation issue to consider in many areas of criminal psychology. Most of the research in this area looks for correlations between measures of different aspects of behaviour (for example, between personality and offending behaviour or between physiological measures and offending behaviour). Such research can only ever show a relationship between two variables and does not

show cause and effect. The relationship may be spurious or there may be a third factor involved that has not been considered. For example, although Raine and Lui have shown a correlation between physiological measures and offending, this does not necessarily mean that physiological factors determine offending. There may be some environmental factor which has affected the physiological functioning of the individual which also contributes to an increased likelihood of offending. In a similar way, Farrington *et al.* have shown a relationship between parental offending and offspring offending, but they have not been able to explain the causal relationship.

The only way to determine a cause-and effect-relationship between two variables is to conduct an experiment where you control one variable and measure its effect on another variable, and for many practical and ethical reasons it is not possible to conduct this kind of research here.

Types of measurement
The three studies reported here collected their data in very different ways. Raine and Lui used a variety of physiological measures, which are reliable measures and unlikely to be strongly affected by demand characteristics, although it is possible that having their heart rate monitored and so on would make people anxious. They also collected medical details about births, which are likely to be highly accurate. They correlated this data with official records of crimes, which are less valid as a measure of offending behaviour. The data are actually records of convictions, not criminal activity, and it is possible that people may have committed crimes that they have not been convicted of or been convicted of a crime that they did not commit. This last comment would also apply to the research conducted by Farrington *et al.*, as their data also came from the Criminal Record Office and so may also be inaccurate. However, as part of the full Cambridge Study, the researchers did ask participants for their self-reports of criminal activity and they state that these were remarkably similar to the official statistics. Finally, Eysenck *et al.* used the Eysenck Personality Questionnaire, a psychometric test that has been developed over a number of years. This test has been well validated and appears to be reliable. However, there are problems with demand characteristics and social desirability bias in any psychometric test (although the EPQ does contain a lie scale designed to pick up contradictory responses which might indicate that someone is lying).

Usefulness/implications
Clearly, determining the causes of criminal behaviour is an extremely useful thing to do. In simple terms, this could lead to the development of prevention programmes for children deemed to be at risk or to treatment programmes for offenders. You will see in the final section of this chapter that the reason many treatment programmes are unsuccessful is that they do not address the causes of the problem. However, there are several problems with this. First, it is highly unlikely that there are single factors that can be identified as the causes of offending behaviours. It is far more likely that offending behaviour is the result of complex interactions between various factors. This might make some of the research in this area reductionist and over-simplistic. Second, there are ethical implications to consider. The type of research conducted by Raine could be applied to the development of 'screening' programmes. It would be very easy for children to be labelled as potential criminals just because they have the type of physiological functioning identified by Raine and Lui or the

personality type of a conman as identified by Eysenck *et al.*, or for children born to convicted parents to be treated very differently by teachers and social workers. This could lead to a self-fulfilling prophecy where children develop the behaviours attributed to them by others. Raine and Lui raise more worrying possibilities, suggesting that the technology exists to change the brain functioning of individuals. This raises serious issues of social control and it is important that the results of research like that of Raine and Lui are treated with caution.

CRIME
Criminal thinking

STUDY 137
Palmer, E., Hollin, C. R., 2000, 'The interrelations of socio-moral reasoning, perceptions of own parenting and attributions of intent with self-reported delinquency', *Legal and Criminological Psychology*, 5, 201–18

| Aim | To consider the relationships between moral reasoning, perceptions of parenting, attribution of intent and self-reported delinquency among young male offenders and non-offenders. |

Aim

To consider the relationships between moral reasoning, perceptions of parenting, attribution of intent and self-reported delinquency among young male offenders and non-offenders.

Method

Correlational, using a variety of psychometric and self-report measures.

Participants

Two groups of participants, all from the Midlands area:
1) 97 convicted male offenders, aged 13–21 years (the offences were typically burglary, car theft, joyriding and assault)
2) 77 non-offenders, aged 12–24 years.

Procedure

There were several different methodologies involved in this study. The researchers were looking for correlations between moral reasoning, perceptions of parenting and attribution of intent with self-reported delinquency. They were also comparing two naturally occurring groups (offenders and non-offenders). Data were collected using a number of psychometric tests which are outlined below:
1) Socio-moral Reflection Measure (short form) – this tests moral reasoning by asking 11 questions, such as whether keeping a promise is important and why (the scores show the level of moral reasoning that the individual has reached)
2) Extracts from Own Perceptions of Parenting (EMBU) – developed in Sweden, this assesses perceptions of parenting (by mother and father separately), including rejection, emotional warmth and overprotection
3) Attribution of Intent – this test investigates the explanations (attributions) that people give for the behaviour of others and includes 12 scenarios, of which four involve someone acting with hostile intent, four involve someone acting with pro-social intent and four are ambiguous (participants have to imagine themselves in the situation and suggest reasons for why people behaved as they did by selecting one of three reasons: 'to be mean or horrible', 'to be helpful or nice' or 'not sure')
4) Self-Reported Delinquency Checklist (SRD) – this is a self-report scale of 46 offences and respondents must indicate which offences they have committed and also how often they were committed.

Results

The SRD results confirm that the groups differed in terms of their offending behaviours. The modal score for the non-offender group was 6, while for the offender group it was 25. Some of the key findings included the fact that offenders were found to have less mature moral reasoning than non-offenders, with the moral reasoning scores of the offender group being typically at the stage where moral decisions are made on the basis of rewards and punishments. It was also found that the offender group perceived both their fathers and their mothers as significantly more rejecting (although the effects were even stronger for paternal rejection). They also made more hostile attributions of intent when the scenarios were ambiguous. Offending scores correlated strongly with paternal rejection and incorrect attributions of hostility and the researchers argue that these two variables are significant predictors for SRD scores.

STUDY 138
Palmer, E. J., Hollin, C. R., 2003, 'Using the Psychological Inventory of Criminal Thinking Styles with English prisoners', *Legal and Criminological Psychology*, 8, 175–87

Aim

The Psychological Inventory of Criminal Thinking Styles (PICTS) is a psychometric test which measures thinking patterns believed to be associated with a criminal lifestyle. The aim of the research was to evaluate the use of this test with English prisoners (research had been conducted previously only in the USA) and consider the implications of this research for practice.

Method

Psychometric testing.

Participants

255 male offenders from six different prisons in England. The most common convictions were for violent offences, burglary, theft and handling stolen goods.

Procedure

All prisoners completed the PICTS scale. This is an 80-item scale measuring the ten thinking styles that have been identified as maintaining a criminal lifestyle. These are:
1) confusion – psychological distress, mental confusion, poor reading ability
2) defensiveness – defensive test-taking style, attempting to conceal difficulties or deficiencies
3) mollification – externalizing blame, rationalizing criminal behaviour
4) cut-off – low frustration tolerance, tendency to remove barriers to criminal behaviour with drugs, or short phrases such as 'fuck it'
5) entitlement – an attitude of privilege or ownership, tendency to misidentify wants as needs
6) power orientation – need for control over others
7) sentimentality – belief that one is really a 'good person' despite involvement in criminal behaviour
8) super-optimism – belief that the negative consequences of crime can be avoided indefinitely
9) cognitive indolence – poor critical reasoning
10) discontinuity – inconsistencies between thinking and behaviour.

Results

There was a correlation between PICTS scores and offending behaviour. Similar results were found in both the USA and UK. Age had an effect on scores, with older offenders having the lower scores. The earlier someone began their criminal career, the higher their scores were, suggesting that their criminal attitudes were deeply entrenched. Similarly, the number of criminal convictions someone had was positively correlated with their scores, suggesting stronger criminal thinking patterns. It was also discovered that PICTS scores showed a significant positive change during a prison sentence. A sub-group of 102 prisoners were tested on arrival in prison and just before release and their scores showed significant improvements in thinking styles. The researchers conclude that PICTS is a sensitive measure that provides useful data and could be employed usefully to measure changes in criminal thinking patterns. However, they state that more research is required to establish norms for use in the UK.

STUDY 139
Yochelson, S., Samenow, S., 1984, *Inside the Criminal Mind*, New York: Random House

Aim
This research is reported in a book rather than a journal article and is an account of the authors' work with mentally ill offenders. The authors claim that it is possible to describe thinking patterns that are common to such offenders.

Method
Interviews.

Participants
255 male offenders resident in a psychiatric hospital in the USA. They had been judged either not guilty by reason of insanity or incompetent to stand trial, or had been referred to the authors by agencies such as the courts, probation services or social services.

Procedure
Each offender was interviewed a number of times as part of the treatment they received in hospital. These interviews were conducted by the authors and were Freudian in nature. These were not standardized interviews and this research could be regarded as a large collection of case studies.

Results
The authors suggest that criminals have quite distinct and erroneous thinking patterns that differentiate them from non-criminals. They conclude that they are essentially in control of their lives and their criminality is the result of choices made from an early age. Further, they suggest that offenders have cognitive processes which lead to a distorted self-image and result not only in criminal choices but also in denial of responsibility.

They describe the criminal personality as characterized by 40 thinking errors, which fall into three broad categories:
1) criminal thinking patterns, which are characterized by fear and, simultaneously, a need for power and control; other features in this category include a search for perfection, lying and inconsistencies or fragmentation of thinking and a lack of time perspective
2) automatic thinking errors, which include a lack of empathy and trust, a failure to accept obligations, a secretive communication style and a perception of themselves as the victim
3) crime-related thinking errors, which include optimistic fantasizing about specific criminal acts with no regard to deterrent factors; this also includes an unrealistic sense of invulnerability.

The authors suggest, therefore, that criminals are not necessarily impulsive, that they have planned and fantasized about their actions and that it is these thinking patterns which need to be confronted in treatment. Yochelson and Samenow claim high success rates in getting offenders to accept that they have a 'criminal personality' and in changing their thinking patterns.

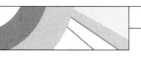

Evaluating research into criminal thinking

Nature/nurture, personality/situation

The research by Palmer and Hollin (2000) suggests that moral reasoning may be related to social/environmental variables such as parenting. This would support a nurture argument as an explanation of moral reasoning. This is in direct contrast to the research reported by Yochelson and Samenow, who argue that criminal behaviour is a choice and that offenders make rational decisions to commit crimes. They do not consider that criminal behaviour can be explained with reference to parents, society, poverty, violent television or any other social/environmental variables. Although they do not explicitly state that this is a nature argument, their arguments reject nurture explanations and certainly would support the 'personality' side of the personality/situation debate. The research by Palmer and Hollin (2003) identifies a variety of different thinking styles that have been associated with criminal behaviour. They do not attempt to explain whether these variables are the result of nature or nurture, although they do report significant changes in thinking styles with age and with time served. These findings would suggest that thinking styles are dependent on nurture or situational influences.

Psychometric measures/ways of collecting data

The research by Palmer and Hollin (2000) used a range of psychometric measures (Socio-Moral Reflection Measure, Extracts from Own Perceptions of Parenting, Attribution of Intent Scale). These are standardized tests and should be both valid and reliable. However, respondents may still give socially desirable answers or may be subject to demand characteristics. In responding to the Delinquency Checklist, there is no way of knowing whether people are telling the truth or not. As a young offender you may not wish to admit to offences for which you had not been caught, for fear of reprisals, or you may say that you have committed many more offences than is actually true for the status that this would give you with your peers. Alternatively, you may simply lie to 'mess up' the research. Palmer and Hollin (2003) used PICTS to assess the thinking styles of offenders. They found a significant correlation between scores with an English population and those with a US population, although more work is necessary to establish norms for an English population. There would appear to be no problems with the reliability or validity of these scales and the researchers claim that it is a highly 'sensitive' measure. Finally, Yochelson and Samenow used Freudian techniques for conducting their clinical interviews and these would not have the same level of reliability or validity as a standardized psychometric test. Data collected in this way are interpreted by the psychiatrist and this may mean that a number of biases are present. Demand characteristics may also play their part here – as an inmate of a psychiatric institution you may have all sorts of reasons for telling the psychiatrist what you think he wants to hear.

Sampling issues

Although Yochelson and Samenow included data from 255 male offenders in their research, they did not have a control group. This means that there is no way of knowing whether the same proportion of the non-offending population may also show these thinking patterns. It has also been suggested that their sample

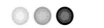

represented a particular sub-group of the criminal population, namely psychopaths, and it has been well documented that psychopaths are highly skilled at manipulation and are able to tell psychiatrists and other professionals exactly what they want to hear. This might suggest that change had not actually taken place. In a similar way, the research by Palmer and Hollin (2003) did not include a control group, although in this case the purpose of the research was to compare the results from English prisoners to the norms already established in US research. In contrast, the research by Palmer and Hollin (2000) compared a sample of young offenders to a comparison group of non-offenders. Matching on all possible variables would be almost impossible in this kind of research, but the inclusion of a comparison group is essential. It could also be argued that in all this research it is only convicted offenders who are studied, and their thinking patterns may differ from offenders who have never been caught as much as they differ from non-offenders. Finally, all the research described here studied males only. This would make generalizing to females very difficult.

Usefulness

The research described in this section is very useful. Both studies conducted by Palmer and Hollin give useful insights into the variables that correlate with moral reasoning and offending scores. Although these are not causal relationships, they do suggest that parenting may be a significant factor in the development of offending behaviour. This would be confirmed by the research conducted by Raine and Lui in the 'Explanations of criminal behaviour' section in this chapter. This might lead to practical suggestions for interventions by social services, but may also generate useful strategies for changing the way people think. From this perspective, the research by Yochelson and Samenow can also be seen to have practical applications. The researchers claim high levels of success in changing the way people think and argue that punishment is essential to rehabilitation. However, it is important to remember that there are a number of reasons why these results may not be accurate. Finally, the research conducted by Palmer and Hollin (2003) may have identified a useful tool for the measurement of change. This would allow accurate measurement of the effectiveness of programmes designed to change the way offenders think.

CRIME
Crime–victim interaction

Aim

The British Crime Survey (BCS) is a huge survey of crime against people living in private households in England and Wales. It is conducted every two years. Comparison with official police statistics reveals some interesting findings.

Method

Survey/interviews.

Participants

The 2000 survey (which measured crime in 1999) used a sample of 19,500 people (and an 'ethnic booster sample' of a further 3,800 people). The sample was randomly selected from the Post Office list of addresses.

Procedure

Participants are questioned in their own homes. Interviewers use a computer program that specifies the questions and the range of permissible answers. All information is given in confidence and no names and addresses are included with the answers. Participants are assured that no information will be passed on and for some of the questions not even the interviewer sees the answers that the participant gives on the computer.

Results

There are numerous results from a survey this size. Some of the key results include:
1) approximately 4.5 times more crime is reported via the BCS than is recorded by the police
2) there was a fall in crime since the last survey (down 13 per cent), with the exception of robbery and theft from the person
3) people are more pessimistic about crime, with one-third believing that the national crime rate had increased when both the BCS and police figures show a decrease
4) fear of crime is higher among those living in high crime areas, those who are recent victims and those who are socially vulnerable (see studies by Donaldson and Beaton *et al.* in this chapter); age, sex and ethnicity all affect levels of fear of crime, with women more worried about all types of crime, older people much more anxious about crime and black and Asian respondents showing higher levels of fear of crime than white respondents.

STUDY 141
Heath, L., 1984, 'Impact of newspaper crime reports on fear of crime: multi-methodological investigation', *Journal of Personality and Social Psychology*, 47, 2, 261–76

| Aim | To examine the effect of newspaper reporting on fear of crime. |

Aim   To examine the effect of newspaper reporting on fear of crime.

Method   Content analysis and telephone interviews.

Participants   62 local newspapers, representing all the local press in 42 US cities for one week. 335 participants were selected randomly and interviewed by phone. Participants were aged 16–83 years.

Procedure   Content analysis – the researchers analysed the crime reports in the newspapers in terms of the proportion of the following:
1) local crime – did the crime occur in the geographical area served by the newspaper or not?
2) random crime – did the report contain any information that suggested that the victim took any action that made him or her more vulnerable? (if not, this is categorized as a random crime)
3) sensationalist crime – was the crime extremely violent or bizarre?
Telephone interviews – these covered newspaper reading habits and various aspects of fear of crime.

Results   Those participants who read newspapers that printed a high proportion of local crime reported higher levels of fear if the crime was described as random or sensationalist. The researchers also conducted a follow-up experiment in which 80 students read fictional accounts of crimes. If these were local and random, participants expressed higher levels of fear. Interestingly, if the crimes were non-local, but random and sensationalist, participants expressed lower levels of fear. The author suggests that this is due to the reports making people feel safer in their own area. This could perhaps be understood using concepts such as Belief in a Just World.

STUDY 142
Donaldson, R., 2003, 'Experiences of older burglary victims', Home Office, Research, Development and Statistics Directorate, Research Findings 198

Aim

People aged over 60 years are statistically far less at risk of burglary than any other age group. However, it is argued that older victims will suffer more severe consequences if they are victims of crimes. This research examined the effects of burglary on victims living in sheltered accommodation.

Method

A natural experiment comparing the naturally occurring variable of domestic burglary.

Participants

Two groups of participants were used:
1) 56 people, aged over 60 years, who had been the victims of domestic burglary (36 females, 20 males, average age = 81 years), all of whom lived in sheltered accommodation (managed by Flintshire Care-Link in North Wales) and received regular visits from a warden
2) a comparison sample of 53 people living in the same sheltered accommodation, but who had not been the victims of burglary (34 females, 19 males, average age = 80 years).

The researcher noted that many other victims were not interviewed as initial contact with relatives suggested that the interviews would be too distressing.

Procedure

Data were collected through semi-structured interviews. These interviews explored general health, circumstances surrounding the burglary, support needed with daily tasks, walking aids, medication and sleeping patterns. Interviews were conducted in the presence of a warden and comments and suggestions were sought from the warden and from relatives.

Results

The results are disturbing. Two years and eight months after the burglary, 11 of the participants had died and a further nine had moved to residential care. In the comparison group, six had died and two had moved to residential care. Relatives typically described the victims' health as deteriorating faster than had been anticipated, victims became increasingly anxious and nervous and many became housebound or spent more and more time with family in order to avoid returning to the sheltered accommodation. Although the sample size is small, these results do suggest that those who had been burgled were more likely to die or become increasingly dependent as a result of their ordeal.

STUDY 143
Beaton, A. *et al.*, 2000, 'The psychological impact of burglary', *Psychology, Crime and Law*, 6, 33–43

Aim	To assess the psychological impact of burglary.
Method	A natural experiment comparing the naturally occurring variable of domestic burglary.
Participants	Two groups of participants were included: 1) 20 victims of residential burglary, aged 23–69 years (12 male, eight female), initially approached via a victim support scheme in Swansea, South Wales 2) a comparison group matched by neighbourhood, age, gender and marital status.
Procedure	Data were collected using questionnaires, which were administered twice: first, one to two weeks after the crime and then, one month later. Questionnaires were administered by trained victim support counsellors.
Results	Victims of crime were more anxious, hostile, depressed, tired, confused and generally more distressed than the controls. One month on there was some improvement in these scores, but these were still significantly different to the comparison group.

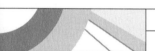

Evaluating research into crime–victim interaction

Strengths and weaknesses of self-report measures

The studies included in this section use a variety of self-report measures, including fixed response questionnaires and semi-structured interviews. Self-report measures have a number of strengths and weaknesses. The strengths are that you are collecting data first-hand, that is, you are actually asking people directly about their experiences, which has more validity than trying to infer something from their behaviour. However, people may lie or exaggerate information, they may be prone to demand characteristics or social desirability bias, or the questions may lead people or force them into predetermined categories of responses. The British Crime Survey suggests that there are 4.5 times as many crimes committed as are reported to the police, which means that either people are not reporting crimes to the police or they are making up a lot of information for the Crime Survey interviewers. Both these explanations may have elements of truth. In the study with older victims of domestic burglary (Donaldson), it is possible that demand characteristics may have accounted for some of the findings. If people are anxious, scared and lonely, it is possible that they would exaggerate their fears in order to keep the interviewer with them for longer or to try to get some additional support. Of course, it is also possible that some people might do the opposite in order to appear more capable than they actually are. The same point may also be true of the victims of crime studied by Beaton *et al.*

Sampling issues

The British Crime Survey uses a very large and randomly selected sample of participants. This means that it is highly likely to be representative of the population of England and Wales. However, you could argue that there are a significant number of people without permanent homes or living on the streets who are likely to be at much greater risk of crime and their voices are not being heard. In comparison, the study by Donaldson uses a very small sample of participants from a single area of Wales. This might make it harder to generalize the findings of this study to other areas, although this research can still be regarded as useful. Further, Donaldson excluded any potential participants who might have found the questioning too distressing and this may further reduce how representative his sample is (although this is the correct ethical procedure). It could also be argued that there might have been differences between his burgled and non-burgled groups which cannot be controlled for, for example, the non-burgled group may have been security-conscious and therefore less likely to be victims of burglary. However, to counter this it could be argued that as they all lived in similar warden-controlled accommodation, security should have been good for all participants. Beaton *et al.* also used a very small sample in their research, although the comparison group were well matched on a number of variables and this increases the reliability of the findings. Finally, Heath used a large sample of participants in her research and they were randomly selected. However, a comparison group of non-local paper readers would have been interesting.

Ethics

The British Crime Survey adheres to all ethical guidelines. No one has to take part, confidentiality is guaranteed and participants can refuse to answer any questions. It could still be argued that this is potentially distressing and some people may be affected by the experience. Donaldson admits that some potential participants were excluded from the study as the interview process was thought to be too distressing. This shows adherence to the guideline Protection of Participants, as does the presence of the warden while the interviews were conducted. However, it could still be argued that the remaining participants in both groups may have been distressed by the interview and perhaps even became more anxious about crime as a result of their participation. This is similar to the research by Beaton *et al.*, which used trained victim support counsellors to conduct the interviews. This would ensure that the appropriate action could be taken if anyone were to become very distressed or reveal information that required further intervention. In conclusion, this type of research does not appear to be highly unethical, but there are a number of issues that should be considered by researchers.

Usefulness

The British Crime Survey is undoubtedly a very useful tool for providing an alternative view of crime to that of the official statistics. The results suggest that many people do not report crimes to the police and this may be because they feel that the police will not be able to do anything to help. The BCS also gives us very useful information about people's fear of crime and their misperceptions of the crime rate. The study by Heath may go some way to explaining why people hold these misperceptions. If you read lots of local crime reports which appear sensationalist or random, your fear of crime will increase. When asked to consider whether crime has increased or decreased in recent years, nearly everyone believes that it has increased when in fact it has decreased. It may be that increased reporting contributes to this, in part. The research by Donaldson highlights the need for increased support for elderly victims of crime who may suffer extreme effects. This research also found that victims were often not kept up-to-date with the progress of their case, in one case not even knowing that the offender had been caught. Elderly people who are very frightened deserve to be told more than anyone when the offender has been caught. Police should be encouraged to visit elderly victims on a regular basis in order to reassure them. The studies by Donaldson and Beaton *et al.* show how people respond to being the victims of crime. Even in relatively minor cases, such as indecent exposure, victims can become increasingly concerned about becoming the victims of other crimes. This could lead to counsellors being trained to reassure people that their fears are understandable, although their likelihood of becoming a victim is no greater than it was before.

STUDY 144

Mokros, A., Alison, L. J., 2002, 'Is offender profiling possible? Testing the predicted homology of crime scene actions and background characteristics in a sample of rapists', *Legal and Criminological Psychology*, 7, 25–43

| Aim | To test the notion that the more similar the background characteristics of offenders, the greater the resemblance in their crime scene behaviour. |

Aim

To test the notion that the more similar the background characteristics of offenders, the greater the resemblance in their crime scene behaviour.

Method

Content analysis.

Participants

100 male British offenders convicted of stranger rape. 61 were assumed to be 'one-off' rapists (one victim statement in police records) and the other 39 were known to have offended more than once (more than one victim statement in police records).

Procedure

Crime scene actions were assessed from victim statements. Where more than one victim statement existed, the earliest and latest were used. In total, 139 victim statements were analysed using content analysis. 28 crime scene actions were coded and these included the use of disguise, the theft of personal property, verbal violence, apologies, use of blindfold, use of weapon and so on.

Information on the offenders' background characteristics, extracted from police files, included age at time of offence, ethnicity, employment status, educational level, marital status and previous criminal record (further analysed by type).

Results

No correlation was found between any of the variables. In other words, rapists who offend in similar fashions are not similar with respect to age, socio-demographic features or criminal records. The authors conclude that the notion of socio-demographic similarity is too simplistic and suggest that future research should consider a framework for offender profiling that is grounded in personality psychology.

STUDY 145
Kocsis, R. N. *et al.*, 2002, 'Investigative experience and accuracy in psychological profiling of a violent crime', *Journal of Interpersonal Violence*, 17, 8, 811–23

Aim

To investigate the hypothesis that investigative experience gives individuals the ability to construct accurate psychological profiles. In other words, will experienced detectives produce better profiles than other groups?

Method

An experiment with independent measures. The independent variable was occupation of participants.

Participants

Six different groups of participants took part in this study, including 31 senior detectives, 12 experienced homicide detectives, 19 trainee detectives, 50 police recruits, 50 police students and 31 undergraduate students majoring in chemistry.

Procedure

All participants were given a case description of an actual solved murder. This included details about the crime scene, sketches and photographs, forensic information and information about the victim. Once participants had read the material they were asked to complete a 45-item multiple-choice checklist, which asked them to assess the offender's physical characteristics, cognitive processes, offence behaviours and social history and habits. The participants were also asked to sign a declaration confirming that they had no prior knowledge of the case.

Results

The results are surprising. The most accurate profiles were produced by the chemistry students, followed by the police recruits and then the experienced senior detectives. This would offer little evidence to suggest that 'investigative experience is the quintessential skill for effective psychological profiling'. Further, as both the chemistry students and the police recruits were studying at higher education level, there is the suggestion that the educational level of these groups may have some bearing on the results and further research into this variable is clearly required.

STUDY 146
Pinizotto, A. J., Finkel, N. J., 1990, 'Criminal personality profiling: an outcome and process study', *Law and Human Behaviour*, 14, 3, 215–33

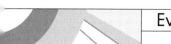

Aim

To compare the accuracy of FBI profilers to detectives, psychologists and students.

Method

An experiment with independent measures. The independent variable was occupation of participants.

Participants

Four trained FBI profilers, six experienced detectives trained in profiling, six experienced detectives without profiling training, six clinical psychologists and six undergraduate students.

Procedure

Each participant was asked to draw up a profile for two crimes. These were solved crimes so that the accuracy of the profile could be assessed. The first crime was a sex offence and the second was a homicide.

Results

Overall, the researchers conclude that the profilers wrote richer profiles with more detail. Specifically, the profilers produced more accurate profiles for the sex offence case, particularly in relation to the sex, age and educational background of the offender. There were no significant differences in the profiles drawn up by each group for the homicide, although the detectives were slightly more accurate in identifying the employment status of the offender and his relationship to the crime scene. Therefore, this study would suggest that there is some evidence to support the notion that profiling training and detective experience lead to the skills necessary to identify offender characteristics.

Evaluating research into offender profiling

Effectiveness of profiling

There are mixed results here and it should be remembered that profiling is a relatively new science and is still being developed. There are a number of different profiling methods in current use (in particular, you should be able to compare the approaches used in the UK with those employed in the USA). It is also difficult to assess the effectiveness of profiling, with some surveys suggesting that profiling adds 'direction' to an investigation rather than directly identifying the offender. What do the studies summarized in this section tell us? First, it is clear that the results found by Kocsis *et al.* contradict the results found by Pinizotto and Finkel. Pinizotto and Finkel found that trained profilers produced more accurate profiles than less experienced police officers or naive participants. This was not a very strong finding, however, and was only confirmed in one of the two cases they used. Surprisingly, Kocsis *et al.* found that it was the chemistry students who produced the most accurate profiles in their research. It is interesting to note that the police officers used in this study were not trained profilers. It is not clear how these findings can be explained, although they clearly indicate the need for further research. The research

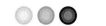

by Mokros and Alison suggests that looking for socio-demographic similarities between offenders is too simplistic and they suggest an approach that is more grounded in personality psychology.

Ecological validity/validity of measurements

Is the type of research we are considering a valid way of testing effectiveness? This is a very difficult question to answer. The studies by Kocsis et al. and by Pinizotto and Finkel both asked participants to read case summaries and then produce a profile. Accuracy was assessed by the number of correct judgements made about the offender's personal characteristics. It may be that some of these judgements are more useful to police than others and it may be that experienced profilers/police are better at identifying certain pieces of information. For example, correctly identifying a number of socio-demographic variables may not be that much help to police, but correctly identifying geographic location or personality characteristics might be. Police surveys have revealed that often it is a single piece of information or the general direction given by the profiler that is useful rather than the number of accurate pieces of information identified. Finally, the investigations by Kocsis et al. and Pinizotto and Finkel were conducted as experimental studies, which may reduce their ecological validity somewhat (although the cases used were real, solved cases), whereas the research by Mokros and Alison was a statistical analysis of a large number of known offenders.

Ethics/ethical implications

The research described here does not raise a large number of ethical issues, although it could be argued that, particularly for the non-police, the case summaries may have been distressing as they included photographs and detailed information of sex crimes and homicide. However, the ethical implications of offender profiling do need to be assessed. The danger in developing a general profile of a serial sex offender, for example, could lead to innocent people being identified as suspects. Remember that if someone matches a profile, this does not mean they are the offender. Mokros and Alison's research highlights the need for more than socio-demographic variables to be included in a profile and this may help to prevent inaccurate accusations. There have been some notable cases in which the use of offender profiling has been heavily criticized (the 'entrapment' of Colin Stagg as a suspect in the murder of Rachel Nickell led to the case being dropped and the police and the profiler being severely criticized for inappropriate behaviour).

Of the three studies described here, one finds no significant correlation between variables typically used in profiles; one finds that experienced profilers write more detailed profiles than non-experienced people; and one finds that chemistry students do better than experienced police. Clearly, the ethical implications of using profiles at present should be considered very carefully indeed.

Usefulness

Despite all the criticism raised above, this research is clearly very useful. It suggests that there is some merit in the use of profiles but that further development of the techniques is still necessary. It is clear that trying to correlate socio-demographic variables with offences is overly simplistic. Profiling should be more firmly rooted in psychological theory and this is a criticism made of the FBI approach to profiling by the UK's leading profiler, David Canter. Canter has also pioneered 'geographic profiling', which has had some notable successes.

The research described here highlights the fact that it is not clear what makes someone a good profiler. It would seem as though experience in police work does not necessarily help, whereas the ability to study at higher education level might. This is an obvious route for further research. If researchers could identify the cognitive processes used by those who create accurate profiles (including psychological variables), this could be incorporated into training programmes. In conclusion, remember that offender profiling is still developing and some of the research here should be seen as reflecting a stage in that development.

CRIME
Police and crime

STUDY 147
Adlam, K. R. C., 1985, 'The psychological characteristics of police officers', in J. R. Thackrah (ed.), *Contemporary Policing*, London: Sphere Reference, cited in Brewer, K., 2000, *Psychology and Crime*, Oxford: Heinemann

Aim	To discover whether British police officers show certain personality traits.
Method	Psychometric testing.
Participants	304 police inspectors, chief inspectors and superintendents at the Police Staff College.
Procedure	Police were tested using the Myers Briggs Type Indicator (MBTI), which was developed from the work of Carl Jung and measures four personality dimensions: 1) Extroversion–Introversion (EI) 2) Sensing–Intuition (SN) 3) Thinking–Feeling (TF) 4) Judging–Perceiving (JP). These four dimensions interact to produce 16 different personality types.
Results	The most common types found in the above sample were ISTJ (Introversion, Sensing, Thinking and Judging), with 38 per cent, and ESTJ (Extroversion, Sensing, Thinking and Judging), with 22 per cent. Both these personality types are described as practical, realistic, unemotional, organized and good administrators. Interestingly, there were few NF (Intuition and Feeling) combinations, which tend to be more imaginative personalities. This would suggest that there are specific personality types in the police force.

STUDY 148
Vrij, A., Mann, S., 2001, 'Who killed my relative? Police officers' ability to detect real-life high-stake lies', *Psychology, Crime and Law*, 7, 119–32

Aim

To examine the ability of police officers to detect deception.

Participants

52 uniformed police officers from the Netherlands (28 male, 28 female, mean age = 31 years, mean length of service = nine years). The majority were tested while attending a lecture on interviewing suspects at a Dutch police school and the remainder were tested at local police stations.

Procedure

The researchers had collected eight short clips from videotaped press conferences where people were asking the general public for help in finding their relatives or the murderers of their relatives. Five clips were of people who had later been convicted of the crime and three clips were assumed to contain no deception. The latter were used as 'filler' items and are not included in the analysis.

The officers had to watch each clip and then indicate:
1) whether they thought the person was lying (yes/no)
2) how confident they were with their decision (1–7 scale)
3) whether they could understand what the person was saying (yes/no) – clips were in English
4) any behavioural cues that prompted their decisions.

Results

Three officers were right 80 per cent of the time, 25 were right 60 per cent of the time, 20 were right 40 per cent of the time, three were right 20 per cent of the time and one officer was wrong on every occasion. By chance, you would expect a score of 50 per cent and the authors claim that this means that those scoring 40 per cent and 60 per cent are therefore scoring at the chance level. This means that 49 of the 52 officers do no better than would have been expected by simply guessing.

Age, length of service, level of experience in interviewing suspects and confidence had no effect on the accuracy scores. However, there was a correlation between level of experience in interviewing suspects and being confident in detecting deception (but not being any more accurate). Finally, men were better at detecting deception than women. The conclusion given here is that detecting deception is a difficult task at which even police officers are not very good.

> **STUDY 149**
> Horselenberg, R., Merckelbach, H., Josephs, S., 2003, 'Individual differences and false confessions: a conceptual replication of Kassin and Kiechel (1996)', *Psychology, Crime and Law*, 9, 1–8

Aim

Kassin and Kiechel (1996) falsely accused students of causing a computer crash and found that 69 per cent of them were willing to sign a false confession, 28 per cent of them internalized the guilt and 9 per cent confabulated detail to support their false beliefs. Kassin and Kiechel claim their study demonstrates how easy it is to elicit false confessions. However, Horselenberg *et al.* point out that there were no negative consequences to signing this false confession and so this study lacks ecological validity. Their study is a replication of Kassin and Kiechel with the addition of negative financial consequences for falsely confessing. They also examine whether personality differences are associated with false confessions.

Participants

34 female undergraduate students with a mean age of 18.6 years. They were told that they were participating in a study to evaluate a new type of keyboard configuration and were paid for their participation.

Procedure

Participants were asked to type characters as they appeared on a computer screen. They were told not to touch the 'shift' key as this would cause the computer to crash and lose all the data. Part way through the test, the computer was made to crash and the experimenter accused the participant of touching the shift key, saying that she had seen it 'with her own eyes' (false incriminating evidence). Then the experimenter asked participants to sign a handwritten confession stating that the data were lost because the participant hit the shift key and would therefore forfeit 80 per cent of the promised fee (negative consequence).

Results

27 out of 34 signed the confession, 14 internalized the guilt and 19 confabulated details. These results show how easy it is to elicit a false confession from someone. Individual differences as tested for with psychometric tests did not appear to have any effect on false confessions. This suggests that false confessions are more likely to be a result of situation than personality.

STUDY 150

Fisher, R. P., Geiselman, R. E., Amador, M., 1989, 'Field test of the cognitive interview: enhancing the recollection of actual victims and witnesses of crime', *Journal of Applied Psychology*, 74, 5, 722–7

Aim

To compare the performance of experienced detectives, pre- and post-training, in cognitive interviewing techniques and to compare their performance post-training with a control group.

Method

A field experiment with repeated measures.

Participants

16 experienced detectives in Florida (seven of whom completed the cognitive interviewing course), whose performance was compared to nine untrained controls.

Procedure

All 16 detectives tape-recorded several interviews. Each detective recorded five to seven interviews over a period of four months and a total of 88 interviews were recorded. These were mainly with victims of commercial robbery or handbag snatching. At the end of this stage the two groups were created. Seven detectives underwent four training sessions of one hour. After training, these seven detectives and six of the remaining nine recorded two to seven interviews. A total of 47 interviews were recorded over seven months. Note: the numbers fell at this stage as several of the original sample were unable to complete the training or the remaining interviews due to work commitments. Interviews were transcribed and scored by independent judges and the number of relevant, factual and objective statements were recorded.

Results

Comparison pre- and post-training – 47 per cent more information was recorded in the post-training interviews and six of the seven detectives in this group did better post-training, with only one doing worse (the authors note that this detective was not using the suggestions given during training).

Comparison of trained group and control group – 63 per cent more information recorded in the interviews conducted by the trained detectives.

These results clearly show the effectiveness of the cognitive interviewing technique over traditional interviewing methods and it could also be suggested that this training is relatively easy to provide.

Evaluating research into police and crime

Personality/situation

The research described here raises several issues associated with the theme of personality/situation and you could also consider the issue of nature/nurture in relation to these studies. The study by Adlam suggests that there are typical personality types within the police force. However, this research did not measure the personality of these individuals before they joined the police force and so it is not possible to determine whether certain types of people join the police or whether

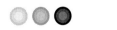

police officers develop these personality characteristics the longer they are in the job (referred to as the 'canteen culture'). Further, you might suggest that as participants completed the questionnaires in a work environment, the situation might have influenced the way in which they responded. The research by Horselenberg *et al.* also raises the issue of personality versus situation. In this research, the authors conclude that it is situation and not personality which determines whether someone makes a false confession. This has obvious implications for the way people are questioned. From the perspective of nature/nurture, you could also examine the other two studies covered in this section. The studies by Vrij and Mann and Fisher *et al.* consider specific skills associated with policing. Vrij and Mann suggest that police do not have the skills associated with identifying deception naturally and the study by Fisher *et al.* suggests that interviewing skills can be learned. This might suggest that there are not specific personality types within the police and that the qualities associated with being a good police officer can be learned (see the section on 'Offender profiling' in this chapter for more on this). However, this does not explain why some people are attracted to police work and others are not. As with most topics in psychology, the answer is likely to be that nature and nurture, as well as personality and situation, interact in complex ways to produce behaviour.

Ecological validity

The study by Vrij and Mann has high ecological validity as it used videos of real press conferences. While you may argue that assessing deception from a video may have lower ecological validity than in a face-to-face situation, it is clearly better to use actual press conference video than to employ actors. In addition participants in this study were tested in normal work-related environments, which would also increase the ecological validity of the study.

In contrast, the study by Horselenberg *et al.* has low ecological validity. It was conducted in laboratory conditions and was an artificially created situation. While the authors may be right in claiming that their study has more realism than the original piece of research by Kassin and Kiechel, the negative consequences were nothing like the potential negative consequences of falsely confessing to a crime. However, this does not detract from the study's conclusion that false confessions are more likely to be due to situational factors than personality factors. The research by Fisher *et al.* was an analysis of real interviews conducted by police officers pre- and post-training in cognitive interviewing techniques and this clearly gives the research a high level of ecological validity. However, drawing conclusions from this research should be done with caution as there are such small numbers of participants involved and demand characteristics may have played a part.

Ethics

The research in this section raises several ethical issues. Probably the biggest ethical issue to consider is deception. Horselenberg *et al.* deceived their participants by insisting that they had done something which they had not. This may have made the participants feel stressed and anxious about the possible repercussions. Clearly, this was necessary to give the study any ecological validity, but the effects of the experience on the participants should be considered carefully when deciding whether a piece of research should go ahead. In their defence, the authors debriefed their participants fully and they did not lose their payment. In contrast, the study by

Adlam raises very few ethical issues as participants were simply asked to complete psychometric tests. The study by Vrij and Mann raises different issues. Participants were not deceived as to the aim of the research, but you could consider the longer-term effects of realizing how poorly you had done at the task of detecting deception. This could have significant effects on your feelings of confidence in relation to your job, and placing people in this type of situation should only be done after careful consideration.

Usefulness

The study by Vrij and Mann highlights the need for training police officers in detecting lies, although the authors do not suggest how this might be achieved. This study also suggests that confidence is unrelated to ability and this may have considerable effects in the courtroom. If an experienced police officer claims that someone is lying, this may carry a lot of a weight with the jury. If the defence presented this research in their evidence, this could seriously undermine the credibility of an authority figure. The Horselenberg *et al.* study is very useful and could be used to demonstrate to police how easy it is to elicit a false confession from someone and hopefully lead to training designed to prevent this. It may also be useful for defence solicitors when they are defending someone who claims that they made a false confession. Fisher *et al.*'s research has obvious implications for training police officers, as all but one of the experimental group elicited more information using the cognitive interview technique. Finally, Adlam's study is more difficult to evaluate. If indeed there are personality differences between police officers and others then this might prove a useful tool for recruitment. However, if these differences are the result of many years in the police force, then psychometric testing may be useful for identifying the traits that lead to successful policing and considering ways of developing these.

CRIME
Psychology of testimony

STUDY 151
Morris, V., Morris, P. E., 1985, 'The influence of question order on eyewitness accuracy', *British Journal of Psychology*, 76, 365–71

Aim
To investigate how question order affects memory. The authors propose that asking participants questions which follow the order of events will lead to better recall.

Method
An experiment with independent measures.

Participants
96 people, aged 18–44 years. This was an opportunity sample of friends and neighbours of the authors. Participants were volunteers and were not paid for participating.

Procedure
Two groups of 48 participants were shown one of two short films, each of which culminated in a chase scene. Two films were used to ensure that effects would generalize beyond a single film sequence. One was a clip of *Starsky and Hutch* and the other was of unfamiliar people. Both clips involved two central characters being pursued, culminating in a chase sequence and the main event. Both clips were approximately five minutes long. Participants were tested at home or in the experimenter's home, either individually or in small groups. All participants were first asked to write a free narrative account of the film. Each group was then subdivided into four equal groups of 12:
1) random order – question order randomized by use of a random number table
2) time sequence – questions asked in order
3) central character – all questions about central character first, followed by the rest in time sequence
4) main event – all questions about the chase asked first, followed by the rest in time sequence.

25 questions were asked on each film. Questions covered a range of detail from what was said by major and minor characters, their appearance and behaviour and other details about the scene.

Results
Free narrative accounts were scored by giving one mark for each correct detail. Less than one incorrect detail per person was recorded. Mean scores were 30.8 (film A) and 28.6 (film B).

Results from the questions showed that time sequence led to the best recall.

Question order	Time sequence	Central character	Main event	Random
% correct	69	66	60	58

STUDY 152
Yuille, J. C., Cutshall, J. L., 1986, 'A case study of eyewitness memory of a crime', *Journal of Applied Psychology*, 71, 2, 291–301

Aim

To examine eyewitness accounts of a real event (as opposed to the numerous laboratory studies of video/staged events).

Method

A case study of a real event (shooting).

Participants

21 witnesses to a gun-shooting incident were interviewed by police after the incident. 20 were contacted later and 13 agreed to be interviewed (refusals included two who had moved away and five who did not wish to 'relive' the experience, one of whom was the victim). The 13 included all the major witnesses, with the exception of the victim and one other who was in prison at the time of the research. Ten were male, three were female and all were aged 15–32 years.

Procedure

The initial police interviews were made available to the researchers and included a verbatim account of the event in the witnesses' words and their responses to a series of questions designed to clarify aspects of the event. The research was conducted with the full cooperation of the Royal Canadian Mounted Police.

Research interviews were conducted four to five months after the event at a time and place chosen by the witness (usually their home or place of work). Interviews were 45–90 minutes and followed the same procedures as the police interview: an account in the witness's own words, followed by questions to clarify earlier points and solicit specific details. The questions included two misleading questions. The first misleading question asked about a broken headlight (following Loftus, 1974). Six of the witnesses were asked if they had seen 'the busted headlight' and the remainder were asked if they had seen 'a busted headlight' (there was no broken headlight). Another similar question was asked about a different coloured panel on the car. These questions were chosen because although the car was in full view of all the witnesses it did not play a major part in the event.

The event was reconstructed from police evidence (photographs, confiscated weapons, witness descriptions etc.) and reports of other professionals attending the scene (ambulance men etc.). Each detail recalled was awarded one point.

Results

The research interview elicited considerably more detail than the police interview:

	Police interview	Research interview
Number of details recalled	649.5	1056.5

Misleading questions had no effect – this is a very different finding to most of the laboratory research conducted into eyewitness testimony. A small amount of information was reported that never happened (2.93 per cent of action details reported to police, 3.23 per cent in research interviews). Again, this is lower than often reported by laboratory research.

STUDY 153
Christie, D., Ellis, H., 1981, 'Photofit constructions versus verbal descriptions of faces', *Journal of Applied Psychology*, 66, 358–63

Aim

To compare the effectiveness of verbal recall of faces with that of photofit techniques used by the police.

Method

An experiment.

Participants

36 participants recruited from a psychology department subject panel (27 women, nine men), aged 29–63 years.

Procedure

There were two stages to this experiment:
1) face recall by description and by photofit construction
2) evaluation (by 'judges') of their respective accuracy.

Participants were shown a target face (six different faces were used) and then were asked to give a verbal description, from memory, followed by the construction of a photofit likeness. Photographs were colour and all showed a young adult male, looking straight ahead; all were photographed in surgical gowns, against the same plain background.

A standard male Caucasian Photofit Kit was used for the construction of the photofit. This divides the face into five features: forehead/hairstyle, eyes, nose, mouth and chin and each feature is selected from a visual index. All participants were tested individually and were shown the target face for 60 seconds. They were then asked to describe the face and all the details were recorded. At the end of the description, if the participant had not mentioned any of the five features listed above they were prompted to do so. This description was used as a general guide to the range of relevant features in the kit. The subject then constructed a visual likeness using the photofit kit. The final likeness was photographed for use in the evaluation stage. Times taken to produce the verbal description and the photofit were recorded.

Accuracy was assessed in two judgement tasks: identification and sorting.

Identification – verbal descriptions were typed on cards (in sets of six, with one description of each photograph), using the feature headings to make them easier to follow. Photofits were also arranged in sets of six, containing one construction of each face. A new array of 24 colour faces of young adult males was constructed, containing the original six faces, with an additional 18 faces.

All this was set up at various points around the university campus. Volunteer 'judges' were sought from students, staff and visitors. Each judge was randomly assigned one set of either verbal descriptions or photofits and asked to identify the target for each description/photofit from the array of 24. Each set of six descriptions/photofits was judged by ten judges (five male, five female) and each description/photofit received a score on a scale of 0–10, depending on the number of people who correctly identified the target face.

Sorting task – two further groups of 16 judges (eight male, eight female) were recruited from a student subject panel. In the first group, each judge was given a pack containing the 36 verbal descriptions, together with the original six photographs. Their task was to sort the descriptions into six groups of six, corresponding with the photographs. The same procedure was followed by judges in the second group for the photofits. The score was the number of times each description/photofit was correctly sorted.

Results

Analysis of both the identification and the sorting tasks suggests a marked superiority for verbal descriptions over photofit constructions. This has obvious implications for police procedure as it suggests that recording a detailed description of the person should be given priority over the creation of a photofit image.

Evaluating research into psychology of testimony

Ecological validity

A great deal of the research conducted in eyewitness testimony is experimental research conducted in the laboratory. The research described above by Morris and Morris is an example of this kind of research (as is the study by Loftus and Palmer that you would have studied during your AS course). Such research tends to lack ecological validity as it differs from a real-life situation in a number of important ways. These include the fact that the participants watch an event on a screen rather than in real life and will probably be expecting to have to answer questions afterwards. Events on television are not as stressful as they would be in real life and all the participants would have been paying attention and viewing the scene from the same distance away. Again, this is unlikely to be the case in real life. If an accident happens, some people may turn round at the sound of the accident or only start watching part-way through and this would obviously affect the accuracy of their testimony. They may also be extremely distressed by what they are viewing, and may be attempting to help in some way. All these factors would have an effect on their later testimony and support the argument that research such as that conducted by Morris and Morris lacks ecological validity. In contrast, the research by Yuille and Cutshall studied a real event and questioned real witnesses. This gives this study much higher levels of ecological validity (although it could also be argued that it means that there are much lower levels of control in this research). Interestingly, this research suggests that people are able to give very accurate reports and are not affected by leading questions. This would shed doubt on the usefulness of laboratory research in this area. Finally, the research by Christie and Ellis is a complex design with many realistic features: participants used genuine photofit technology and naive participants attempted to match the descriptions/photofits to the photographs. However, this was not a real event – participants were expecting to have to recall the face and they would not have had the same emotional involvement in what they were doing as might a witness to an actual crime.

Sampling

The study by Morris and Morris used an opportunity sample of friends and neighbours. This is likely to be a biased sample in a number of ways. It is unlikely that you would get a representative sample in this way and friends and neighbours may be more likely to respond to demand characteristics and try to behave in the way they think the experimenters want them to. Generalizing from these results would have to be done with reservations. In contrast, the study by Christie and Ellis recruited participants from a subject panel, which would give a wider variety of ages and occupations (and may allow researchers to select a representative sample), but may also be biased as all the participants are those who have expressed an interest in volunteering for psychological research and this may have an effect on the way they respond. It has been suggested, for example, that volunteers are slightly more compliant than non-volunteers. The sample used by Yuille and Cutshall could also be discussed here. The participants here were real witnesses to a real crime, which had taken place four or five months previously. The researchers were able to track down a large proportion of the original witnesses, but some crucial ones were not prepared to take part in the research. This may have implications for the validity of this research.

Ethics

Is it ethical to show people films that may distress them? If you had been involved in an accident or a similar type of situation, would you want to be reminded of this? The research by Morris and Morris showed participants video footage that was unlikely to be very distressing (but there may have been individual differences here). Research into real cases, such as that conducted by Yuille and Cutshall, raises different ethical issues. The participants in this study had already experienced the event and it may have been distressing for them to discuss it again. Arguably, the researchers followed the guidelines by not pressurizing people to take part and it may be assumed that those who did participate were happy to do so. However, they should ensure that any follow-up help, such as counselling, was made available to the participants if they found the research more distressing that they had anticipated.

Usefulness/practical applications

Research into areas of applied psychology should generate useful findings and the research into testimony is no exception. You could consider whether research that is low in ecological validity can be useful or not. Loftus and Palmer (AS course) and Morris and Morris showed that participants are strongly affected by leading questions and question order. This would generate the useful suggestion that police and other interviewers take care to avoid leading questions and follow 'event order' when questioning witnesses. Recent developments in cognitive interviewing would support these claims. However, it could also be argued that research by Yuille and Cutshall would suggest that laboratory research does not reveal how witnesses respond in real-life cases. This might lead you to the suggestion that laboratory research in this area has only a limited application and more research into real cases is necessary. The research by Christie and Ellis has some surprising results, demonstrating that people's written descriptions were of more use than their photofit images in identifying the target face. This could be used to argue that police should not rely entirely on photofit images and should pay at least an equal amount of attention (if not more) to a witness's description.

STUDY 154
Stewart, J. E., 1985, 'Appearance and punishment: the attraction–leniency effect in the courtroom', *The Journal of Social Psychology*, 125, 3, 373–8

Aim	To look for a correlation between the attractiveness of a defendant and the severity of the punishment awarded. The authors are predicting a negative correlation: that is, as the attractiveness of the defendant increases, the severity of punishment will decrease.
Method	Observation.
Participants	60 criminal trials were observed in Pennsylvania, USA. The defendants were a range of ages (56 male, only four female). 27 were black, three were Hispanic and 30 were white. Eight observers were used (all white) and each was given a standard rating form. Each trial was observed by at least two observers.
Procedure	Observers rated the defendants on a range of scales. These included physical attractiveness, neatness, cleanliness and quality of dress. These four items were combined to produce an attractiveness index. Several other ratings were also carried out and the most important of these was posture.
Results	No significant correlation was found between race and the attractiveness index. The researchers found a high level of agreement between the different raters. However, the attractiveness index was negatively correlated with punitiveness, that is, the less attractive the defendants were judged to be, the more severe their punishment. The fifth item, posture, also showed this negative correlation.

STUDY 155

Pennington, D. C., 1982, 'Witnesses and their testimony: effects of ordering on juror verdicts', *Journal of Applied Social Psychology*, 12, 4, 318–33

Aim

To examine whether there is a primacy effect or a recency effect in relation to witness testimony. Much previous research had found recency effects, demonstrating that the later information had the most powerful effect on jury decisions. However, Pennington claims that such research does not adequately simulate a real courtroom and predicts that the results will be different in his simulated courtroom procedure.

Method

A simulated courtroom procedure. This is an experimental design with independent measures.

Participants

192 undergraduate students (96 male, 96 female). All were eligible for jury service in the UK and any that were not were excluded from this study.

Procedure

Some participants heard witnesses give 'guilty' testimonies first and others heard witnesses give 'innocent' testimony first. Overall, each participant was exposed to exactly the same material, but in a different order.

Results

The group that heard the guilty witnesses first produced more guilty verdicts than the other group. They were also more confident in their judgements. This suggests strong primacy effects in courtroom decision making.

STUDY 156
Broeder, D., 1959, 'The University of Chicago jury project', *Nebraska Law Review*, 38, 744–60

| Aim | To examine the effect of information being ruled inadmissible by a judge. Is it possible that for at least some jury members, being told to disregard information makes it even more important? |

Method An experiment.

Participants The research was conducted at the University of Chicago Law School. The individuals who participated were actually on jury service at the time and agreed to serve on experimental (mock) juries formed by the researchers.

Procedure These experimental juries listened to tapes of evidence from previous trials and were asked to deliberate as if they were hearing the case. In one part of this research, 30 experimental juries listened to the case of a woman who was injured by a car driven by a careless male driver.

Results When the driver said that he had liability insurance, the jurors awarded the victim an average of $4000 more than when he said he had no insurance ($37,000 versus $33,000). This suggests that juries make larger awards to victims if an insurance company will have to pay.

The second finding is the more interesting one. If the driver said he was insured and the judge ruled that evidence inadmissible (directing the jury to disregard it), the average award to the victim increased to $46,000.

In other words, when juries learned that the driver was insured, they increased the damage payment by $4000. When they were told they must officially disregard this information, they used it even more, increasing the damage payment by $13,000. This research is supported by many other social psychological studies, which demonstrate that banned information acquires greater salience.

STUDY 157
Ross, D. F. *et al.*, 1994, 'The impact of protective shields and videotape testimony on conviction rates in a simulated trial of child sexual abuse', *Law and Human Behaviour*, 18, 5

Aim

To examine the effects on conviction rates if children give evidence in sexual abuse cases in court or with a protective shield or via videotape.

Method

An experiment.

Participants

300 students (150 male, 150 female). The majority were white and middle class.

Procedure

Simulation of a sexual abuse trial. This was based on actual court transcripts and videotaped in a real courtroom using legal professionals. The video lasted two hours.

The independent variable was the way in which the child (a ten-year-old girl) gave her evidence. In condition 1 she gave her evidence in court, directly confronting the defendant. In Condition 2 she gave her evidence in the courtroom, but with a protective shield. In Condition 3 she gave evidence on video.

Study 1 – in the first study, the participants watched the whole video and were then asked to judge the guilt of the defendant.

Results

The type of testimony had no effect on conviction rates, although there was a tendency for females to return more guilty verdicts than males.

Type of testimony	% guilty verdicts	% not guilty verdicts
Open court	51	49
Protective shield	46	54
Video	49	51

Procedure

Study 2 – in the second study, the same procedure was followed with a new sample of 300 students. However, the video was stopped immediately after the child gave her evidence and the participants were asked to make their judgement at this point.

Results

When evidence was given in open court, more convictions were returned than in the protective shield and video conditions.

However, it is the effect on the final decision that is crucial and this study demonstrates that the use of video or protective shields does not significantly reduce the likelihood of a conviction.

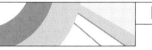

Evaluating research into psychology of the courtroom

Ecological validity

The study by Stewart has high ecological validity as this was an observation of real trials. The observers were rating real defendants in real courtrooms. This is in contrast to numerous studies in this area which simply ask people to read a summary of a trial and then state how they would vote. Pennington's study is an exception to this as it has much higher ecological validity than many other courtroom studies because it followed the exact procedures of a courtroom. However, participants made independent judgements about the guilt of the defendant rather than discussing this in a jury and, once again, they know that it is not a real case and that the decisions they make have no real consequences. These differences are important and it is highly unlikely that participants respond in the way they would if they were on a real jury. Ross *et al.*'s study also has good ecological validity as it was based on a real case, filmed in a real courtroom and used legal professionals as actors. However, participants watched this trial on video and this may have significantly affected the realism of the experience. In fact, this means that all participants watched evidence on video and some watched a video of someone giving evidence on a video, which may have affected not only the ecological validity of the research, but also the conclusions that can be drawn. Finally, Broeder's study is more difficult to assess. Participants listened to tapes of evidence which would have low ecological validity, but the fact that they were serving on juries at the time may have made the whole experience more realistic to them and this may have affected their responses.

Sampling

There are several issues that could be discussed under the heading of sampling; these include the size of the sample, the choice of participants and the effects of these on the generalizability and representativeness of the sample. The sample sizes of the studies described above vary. The four experimental studies used between 192 participants (Pennington) and 300 participants (Ross *et al.*). All these samples are of a size that may be classed as adequate or better, but there are other factors to consider. Pennington and Ross *et al.* used undergraduate students for their studies and there are many ways in which this would not be considered representative of society as a whole. There are possible race, class, age and general life experiences to consider. Pennington points out that the sample he selected were all eligible for jury service and this does increase the representativeness of this sample to an extent. The sample used by Broeder has definite advantages over the other experimental studies as all these participants were actually serving on real juries at the time of the study. This would mean that they had all gone through the very rigorous process of jury selection that is common in the US. This would also create greater ecological validity for this study. It is worth considering the sample size used by Stewart also. This study observed 60 trials, which is a relatively small number to generalize from. Further, this sample included only four females, although it did include a range of different races.

Ethics

Psychological research should protect participants from harm or distress. It is possible that some of the details of the crimes considered by this research may have distressed the participants. In particular, the study by Ross *et al.* may have been very distressing for many participants and it is not clear whether any screening took place to exclude participants who had been victims of abuse, or indeed whether they were told of the content of the trial before they agreed to participate. A related ethical issue could also relate to the process of filming the mock trial. This may have been a distressing experience for the child actor involved. The issue of consent and observation might also be considered in relation to the study by Stewart. It could be argued that a courtroom is a public place and that it is therefore appropriate for defendants to be observed in this way, but you could also argue that observations like this one invade a person's privacy and should not be conducted.

Usefulness

The study by Stewart would have many useful applications for people who have to appear in court. Not only do the results show that appearing neat, clean and well dressed is likely to reduce your sentence, it could also be suggested that the same effect may be found for witnesses. Witnesses scoring high on attractiveness index measures are likely to be perceived more favourably by jurors and their evidence taken more seriously. Pennington's study is very useful as it contradicts many earlier research studies, which found strong recency effects. Pennington argues that this is due to the unnatural conditions used in such research. This relates to the issue of ecological validity discussed above. Results from research with low ecological validity should be applied cautiously. Pennington's research could also suggest useful strategies for lawyers deciding how to present evidence and may also highlight biases in the standard courtroom procedure, which presents prosecution evidence first. The study by Broeder would also suggest that lawyers could turn the inadmissibility of evidence to their own advantage. It would appear that it is worth stating something that you know will be ruled inadmissible as it will in fact assume greater weight when jurors are making their final decisions. Finally, Ross's study has many useful applications as it suggests that the use of protective shields/video does not put the defendant at a higher or lower risk of conviction than testifying in open court and this means that the experience of court for child witnesses can be made much safer and less traumatic.

> ## STUDY 158
> Farrington, D. P., Ditchfield, J., Howard, P., Jolliffe, D., 2002, 'Two intensive regimes for young offenders: a follow-up evaluation', Home Office, Research, Development and Statistics Directorate, Research Findings 163

| Aim | To test the impact of demanding, highly structured regimes on reconviction rates two years after release. |

Method

This is similar to a natural experiment, comparing the reconviction rates following two different regimes.

Participants

Young male offenders, aged 18–21 years, with approximately six months of their sentence left to serve, assessed as suitable for open prison (no previous escape or sex offences) and considered mentally and physically able to cope with the regime.

Procedure

Two institutions were studied. Both were styled on US boot camp regimes.
1) Thorn Cross High Intensity Training Centre (opened July 1996): this centre offers a highly structured, 25-week programme of activities (16 hours a day), including military drilling.
2) Colchester Young Offender Institution (opened in February 1997): this has a 26-week programme based on the military regime and ethos at the Military Corrective Training Centre at Colchester.

The expected reconviction rates were calculated and these were compared to actual reconviction rates two years after release. Reconviction rates were also compared to a control group of young offenders in standard regime institutions.

Results

Thorn Cross HIT – although there were no significant differences in reconviction rates, the Thorn Cross experimental group took longer to reoffend and committed significantly fewer crimes. The cost of the regime was more than recouped by the savings made by the smaller number of crimes committed.

Colchester – although the Colchester experimental group committed slightly fewer crimes than the control group, their crimes were more costly and the authors estimate that this regime was not cost-effective. However, the Colchester experimental group had significantly more positive attitudes towards staff and other inmates and were more hopeful about the future.

The authors conclude that the success of the Thorn Cross regime in reducing reconviction rates was probably due to the education, employment, mentoring and through-care components rather than the drilling and physical training components, as the Colchester regime, which emphasized physical activities, was not successful.

STUDY 159

Friendship, C., Blud, L., Erikson, M., Travers, R., 2002, 'An evaluation of cognitive behavioural treatment for prisoners', Home Office, Research, Development and Statistics Directorate, Research Findings 161

Aim   To evaluate the success of cognitive behavioural treatments for prisoners.

Method   This is a type of field experiment. The experimental group took part in the Cognitive Skills Programme and the control group did not. Reconviction rates were compared.

Participants   670 adult male offenders serving a custodial sentence of two years or more and who voluntarily participated in one of two cognitive skills programmes run by HM Prison Service between 1992 and 1996.

Procedure   The programme is referred to as the Cognitive Skills Programme and consists of two multi-modal programmes focusing on correcting maladaptive or faulty thinking patterns which have been linked with offending behaviour. The programmes were Reasoning and Rehabilitation (36 sessions totalling 72 hours) and Enhanced Thinking Skills (20 sessions totalling 40 hours). Taken together, the aims of the programme are:
1)   self-control (thinking before acting)
2)   interpersonal problem-solving skills
3)   social perspective taking
4)   critical reasoning skills
5)   cognitive style
6)   understanding the rules which govern behaviour.
Reconviction rates were compared to a group of 1801 male offenders who had not participated in any programme.

Results   The results showed a significant drop in reconviction rates. Reconviction rates after two years were up to 14 per cent lower than the comparison groups. The authors suggest that, based on the number of prisoners expected to complete a cognitive skills programme in 2002–3, this reduction represents almost 21,000 crimes prevented.

STUDY 160
Sugg, D., Moore, L., Howard, P., 2001, 'Electronic monitoring and offending behaviour –
reconviction results for the second year of trials of curfew orders', Home Office, Research,
Development and Statistics Directorate, Research Findings 141

Aim To examine the effectiveness of electronic-monitoring curfew orders.

Method This is similar to a natural experiment. Reconviction rates for those who were tagged were compared to predicted reconviction rates and also to reconviction rates of those who were given community service orders.

Participants 261 offenders from Norfolk, Manchester and Reading who had been given curfew orders with electronic monitoring between July 1996 and June 1997 (the second year of the 'tagging' trials). 91 per cent of the sample were male and most were in their mid- to late twenties. Typical offences were theft, burglary and driving offences. The average number of previous convictions was eight.

Procedure The probability of the sample being reconvicted was calculated using OGRS2. This is a Home Office algorithm which predicts the probability of an offender being reconvicted, based on age, criminal history and time in youth custody. This suggested that the sample could be considered to be of medium to high risk of reconviction. The analysis suggested 67 per cent would be reconvicted at the end of two years. This prediction was then compared with actual reconviction rates.

Results 72.8 per cent (190/261) had been reconvicted within two years and 166 of those were reconvicted within one year. The researchers also compared the reconviction rates of the tagged group with a matched comparison group of offenders sentenced to community service orders (the most likely alternative had tagging not been available). There was no significant difference between these two groups. 160 of the 261 also had community service orders running in addition to the tagging. There was also no significant difference between this sub-group and the remaining 101 offenders in terms of reconviction rates.

The authors conclude that curfew orders have no significant effect on offending behaviour and argue that this is because such orders do not address the real problems. However, they cite evidence to suggest that curfew orders can be useful in conjunction with other programmes, such as cognitive behavioural programmes, not least because they tend to increase attendance on such programmes.

STUDY 161

Honess, T., Charman, E., 1992, 'Closed circuit television in public places: its acceptability and perceived effectiveness', Police Research Group Crime Prevention Unit Series, Paper 35, Home Office Police Department

Aim	

This report examines a range of issues to do with public perceptions of CCTV. The research was conducted in 1991, when CCTV was relatively uncommon. For the purposes of this summary, we will just consider the issues of perceived acceptability and effectiveness.

Method	

A large-scale attitude survey, with most questions using Likert-type scales.

Participants	

798 people approached randomly on the streets of four large cities (Birmingham, Cardiff, Bristol and Coventry). Managers of sites with CCTV (such as car parks and shopping centres) were also asked how effective they thought CCTV had been.

Results	

The majority of respondents were aware of at least one site with CCTV and this was most commonly in building societies. There was a generally positive response to the installation of CCTV, although concerns were raised that systems might be abused and that CCTV represented a gradual erosion of our civil liberties. CCTV was seen as more acceptable in sites such as shopping centres and car parks than out in the street. Respondents also had some concerns about who should be allowed to install CCTV and who should be allowed access to the tapes. However, most respondents agreed that CCTV did make them feel safer.

Site managers tended to regard CCTV as part of their general management, allowing them to monitor traffic flow, deliveries and so on, and listed crime prevention as only one function of CCTV. The general public, on the other hand, tended to regard CCTV as having crime detection as its primary purpose. Managers commented on the increased security (not possible to cover such a wide area with security staff, so CCTV represented large cost savings) and some mentioned advantages such as reduction in costs for replacing broken windows or other incidents. However, most comments were more general and included public reassurance and the creation of a safe and secure environment.

The authors conclude that 'public acceptance is based on limited and partially inaccurate knowledge of the functions and capabilities of CCTV systems in public places'. They suggest that there is a need for guidelines and procedures that will ensure the effectiveness of CCTV, minimize threats to civil liberties and make possible an informed public acceptance.

Evaluating research into punishments and treatments

Effectiveness of treatments and punishments

The research presented here is generally positive about the effectiveness of the treatments described. Although the intensive regimes described by Farrington *et al.* are not as effective as you might imagine, this research does highlight education, employment, mentoring and through-care as the variables which ensure success. Interestingly, the physical activities which are a key component of such intensive regimes appeared not to have the desired effect without the variables mentioned above. Friendship *et al.* demonstrate a highly effective outcome from their Cognitive Skills Programme, with reconviction rates after two years significantly lower than a control group who did not participate in any programme. However, electronic monitoring was not found to be successful, with no significant differences between the expected reconviction rates without electronic monitoring and the actual rates. However, neither is it unsuccessful, as it produces similar results to other punishments and is presumably very much cheaper. The authors suggest that using electronic monitoring in conjunction with other programmes may be successful and this is discussed below.

Research methods/measuring effectiveness

It is difficult to conduct research in this area. All research is conducted in the field, as clearly it would not be possible to conduct laboratory-style research in this area. Researchers then have a choice about how to design the research. Farrington *et al.* chose a comparison between two regimes, with effectiveness measured by reconviction rates, Friendship *et al.* included a 'no treatment' control group and also used reconviction rates as a measure of success. Sugg *et al.* took a slightly different approach, with actual reconviction rates being compared to predicted conviction rates. These studies obviously all have the problem of confounding variables and lack of control, but the main issue we shall discuss here is the use of reconviction rates as a measure of success. There are a number of problems with reconviction rates: first, they are not a measure of reoffending. It is possible that people are committing crimes that they are not being convicted for and it is also possible that, due to stereotyping, people are being convicted of crimes they have not committed. It might also be possible that some of these treatments are not stopping people from reoffending, but are making them less likely to be caught (or less likely to be convicted if they are caught). People may also reconvict because they return to the same environment they lived in before, with the same peer group and all the same reasons for committing crimes. Without increased employment or educational opportunities, it is highly likely that reoffending will occur. This does not necessarily mean that the treatment or punishment has had no effect, rather that other factors also come into play. For example, cognitive therapy may change the way someone thinks, but not their behaviour. Finally, reconviction rates do not tell you whether people are committing the same crimes again or different ones, whether these are less serious or more serious and so on. There have also been criticisms of the Home Office statistical formula (OGRS2), as used by Sugg *et al.* This predicts the likelihood of someone reoffending, based on age, criminal history and time in youth custody. This excludes a number of other individual factors, which may play a part.

Ethics and ethical implications

As most of this research takes the form of natural experiments there are no major ethical issues raised by the research itself. You could suggest that deliberately leaving one group 'untreated' could be harmful to them and should not be done solely for the purposes of research. You could also consider whether the testing of treatments and punishments on prisoners is ethical, as presumably they have no choice about participating. This raises issues of civil liberties, privacy and confidentiality. Honess and Charman raise concerns about who should be allowed to use CCTV and who should have access to the tapes. Despite these ethical reservations, however, most respondents in this survey agreed that CCTV made them feel safer, and since this research was conducted, the use of CCTV has become more and more widespread. You could also consider whether some of the actual treatments and punishments are ethical in themselves. Are some aspects of the intensive regimes too harsh for young offenders? Is it right to attempt to change the way someone thinks? Does the use of electronic tagging raise civil liberties issues? These are difficult questions to answer and need to be considered in the light of crime reduction and public safety.

Usefulness
Possibly the most useful conclusion to be drawn from this research is that, in most cases, treatments are more effective than punishments, and treatments which include cognitive components as well as employment opportunities are the most effective. As more research is done and more psychological treatments are developed, hopefully we will see a reduction in the cycle of reoffending that is currently so common. Honess and Charman also highlight the usefulness of CCTV, not only in reducing crime but also in reducing people's fear of crime, which could have a significant effect on the way in which public spaces are used. Finally, the development of alternative ways of measuring effectiveness could be a useful direction for practitioners. Finding the reasons for reoffending will help develop better and more effective treatment programmes.

See also...

Studies 96, 102, 111 and 112.

COURSEWORK

Coursework requirements are subject to change. At the time of writing (spring 2004), OCR A2 students were required to complete two pieces of coursework: a practical report (1400 words) and an assignment (1000 words). Together these two pieces of coursework are worth one-third of the marks for your A2 assessment (and one-sixth of the marks for your whole A level). This coursework is sent to an external examiner for marking.

Some students find the relatively low word limits difficult. It is crucial that you stick to these limits, as failing to be concise can cost you a lot of marks. If you are irritated at having to cut down your work, remember that you are developing a useful examination skill. If you are able to identify the key points in research and describe and evaluate these concisely (without waffling!) then your examination answers will be of a very high standard.

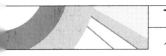

The practical report

This can be on any area of psychology that you choose, but you would be well advised to select a research question relevant to your A2 course. You will need to identify relevant background research, construct a specific research question, select an appropriate method for collecting data, analyse the data and draw conclusions. You will also need to evaluate the research you have carried out.

Currently the word limit for the practical project is 1400 words and going over this limit means that your work will be penalized.

Checklist for the practical report

Remember, before you can conduct the practical report you must have ethical approval for your work. OCR does not allow you to conduct experimental research with children, manipulate any negative variables (such as aggression) or put participants into situations where they are deceived or may be upset or embarrassed. Your teacher or lecturer will have full details of the ethical guidelines provided by OCR and will give you the form to complete. Do not begin your practical work until the proposal has been approved. You will need to submit the signed proposal form with your work.

Make sure your report contains the following:

Title
This should be clear and simple and reflect what the research is about. Something like 'The effect of organization on memory' is fine.

Abstract
An abstract can be regarded as a summary of the whole report. If someone reads your abstract they should understand the aim, method, findings and conclusions of the research. Make sure you cover each of these aspects very briefly (writing one sentence on each of these would ensure that you have covered everything). You will

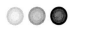

probably find that it is easier to write your abstract once all the other sections of the practical report are complete.

Background/introduction

In this section, you need to show how your research fits into a psychological context. This means describing a piece of relevant research (or theory) which has led you to your hypothesis. For example, if you wanted to investigate the effect of question type or questioning style on eyewitness memory, you might outline the research by Loftus and Palmer (AS course) or Morris and Morris (this volume). You should explain the research clearly and then explain how this research led you to the hypothesis that you are predicting.

Aims/hypotheses

Most research will include a formal hypothesis and a null hypothesis. The only exceptions might be observational research or some type of survey research, where you have a more general aim. Ensure that your hypothesis is clearly stated and includes both variables. Also ensure that you have stated a null hypothesis (which predicts 'no effect').

Methodology

You should include details of all the following points where they are appropriate:
1) state the design of the study and the reasons for the selection of that design
2) describe the sample and the sampling method
3) describe the materials/apparatus that were used in the study (and the reasons for choosing them, if appropriate)
4) explain the procedure clearly, including any standardized instructions given to participants and any controls used in the study
5) explain how the variables were measured and how the data will be analysed
6) give details of any ethical issues you had to consider.

This may sound like a lot of information to include, but it is important that someone reading a report of psychological research understands exactly how you conducted the research and that someone else should be able to replicate the study.

Results

The important thing to bear in mind when reporting your results is that the examiner will be trying to assess how well you understand the results. There is no point producing half a dozen complex graphs on a computer and simply including them in your report. If you do not describe the graphs and point out what they show, you may as well leave them out.

Keep tables and graphs simple (go for summaries of results rather than large graphs that show every individual score) and ensure they are correctly labelled. Explain what the table/graph shows, even if it is obvious.

If you have conducted a statistical analysis of your results (and you should if your data allows you to), ensure that you have used the right test and that you can explain why you used this test (e.g. you would justify using a Mann-Whitney test by explaining that the data was of ordinal level and the design was independent measures). Present the results of the analysis in the results section and put the calculations in an appendix.

Finally, ensure you summarize the key findings at the end of this section and state whether the hypothesis or the null hypothesis has been supported.

Discussion

There are a number of areas that you need to cover in your discussion. You can use subheadings if you wish. Start by stating the results again. This might be a simple sentence that states the decision you have made about the hypothesis. Follow this by a few sentences relating these results back to the material you covered in the background/introduction (e.g. Do your results agree or disagree with those findings? Do they add anything to the original findings? If they are different, why might they be different?).

Identify a few strengths and weaknesses of the research that you have conducted. It is tempting to simply list everything you can think of, but it is better to concentrate on one or two key issues. The more specific these are to your research, the better. For example, you would get good marks for a comment about the actual measure you used and how this might be improved, but fewer marks for a more general point about testing more people. You can also make some suggestions here for further research that could be conducted in the area of your investigation.

References

A complete set of references must be included at the end. This should be presented in the standard format and in alphabetical order.

Books are referenced as follows:

Lintern, Fiona, Stapleton, Merv and Williams, Lynne, 2004, *Study Guide for OCR Psychology: A2 Level*, London: Hodder and Stoughton.

Journal articles are referenced as follows:

Mokros, Andreas and Alison, Laurence J., 2002, 'Is offender profiling possible? Testing the predicted homology of crime scene actions and background characteristics in a sample of rapists', *Legal and Criminological Psychology*, 7, 25–43.

If you are giving the reference for a piece of research that you read about in a book, you should give the reference as follows:

Mokros, Andreas and Alison, Laurence J., 2002, 'Is offender profiling possible? Testing the predicted homology of crime scene actions and background characteristics in a sample of rapists', *Legal and Criminological Psychology*, 7, 25–43, cited in Lintern, Fiona, Stapleton, Merv and Williams, Lynne, 2004, *Study Guide for OCR Psychology: A2 Level*, London: Hodder and Stoughton.

This may seem very long-winded, but it makes it clear to the reader/examiner that you didn't read the original article. If the book authors gave an inaccurate portrayal of the original research, you are making it clear where you got your information from.

If your information came from a website you should also reference this, giving as much detail as you can and including the date when you accessed the information.

Appendices

Appendices are where you put information that the reader might wish to refer to. Typically this might include a copy of your materials (word lists, questionnaires etc.). You need to include only one copy of this sort of information rather than each participant's completed questionnaire. You might also include raw data and the calculation of your statistical analysis. Make sure that you refer the reader to the appendix so they know the information is there.

Final checks

Read your report through and check for mistakes. Check that you have not exceeded the word limit (references and appendices are excluded from this) and make adjustments if necessary. If you can, give your work to someone else to read and ask them to tell you if they understand it. Sometimes another person can point out errors or unclear aspects of the work which you have missed. Make sure that your teacher or lecturer sees the report in its draft stages and that you take note of any suggestions they make.

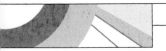

The assignment

This piece of work involves the selection of an appropriate source article (usually from a newspaper or magazine) which raises psychological issues. You will need to write a short report showing how psychological theories and research can be used to help understand the issues raised in the article. Currently the word limit for the assignment is 1000 words and going over this limit means that your work will be penalized.

Checklist for the assignment

Selecting a source article

The best source articles come from magazines and newspapers. They will discuss an issue that has some psychological content, although the article will not provide the psychological analysis. For example, an article discussing crime may raise issues about why people commit crimes, criminal thinking and the effectiveness of punishment. An article about football violence may raise issues of aggression, conformity to group norms and prejudice. The best articles to use are ones that simply raise these issues without making any attempt to explain them in psychological terms (or make unsubstantiated assumptions, such as saying 'crime is all the fault of poor parenting').

Although you can pick an article on anything at all, it may be better to find one which raises issues related to the topics you have studied at AS or the topics you are studying at A2. Once you have selected the source article you will need to identify relevant research. If you are able to do this using your AS/A2 textbooks (and hopefully this book will provide an excellent source of research evidence!) then your task will be made easier. Of course, it is perfectly acceptable to select an article on a topic that you have not studied, but you will need to ensure that you have access to books that will provide you with the relevant evidence.

There are three key sections to your finished assignment. These are as follows:

Assumptions or issues

You need to identify three issues or assumptions raised by your source article. These need to be clearly set out and their relevance to the article fully explained. You might do this by quoting a relevant phrase from the article. The examiner will not work on your behalf here and will be looking to see that you have explained why these issues are important. The examiner will also be looking for evidence that you understand the links between the issues that you have identified and psychology. If you explain briefly which evidence you are going to apply to the issue and why, then you will gain marks here.

Evidence

Briefly describe the evidence you have chosen. There is a strict word count for this assignment so you need to develop your summarizing skills. You don't want to use up all the word count on description as there are other skills you must demonstrate. Once you have presented the evidence, you need to explain clearly why and how it is relevant to the issue/article. Again, the examiner is looking for evidence of understanding here: the more clearly you can link the source and the psychology the better.

Suggestions

For each of the issues you have selected, make a specific practical suggestion about how psychology could be used to help (e.g. Is there a practical intervention that could reduce a problem? Is there information available from psychological research that aids our understanding of the issue? Is there further research that needs to be conducted in order to gain greater understanding?). Also you could evaluate (briefly) your suggestions by commenting on how easy they might be to put into practice, how likely they might be to succeed or what factors might prevent them from succeeding.

References

As with the practical project, each piece of evidence should be referenced fully. See above for examples of how to do this.

Final checks

Read your assignment to yourself. Have you used psychological terms and concepts appropriately? Is it clear to the reader that you understand these concepts? Have you made the links between the source (issues) and the article as clear as you possibly can? Finally, ask someone else to read your assignment. Do they understand the points you are trying to make? Do they need to ask you for additional information? Do they agree with the arguments you are putting forward? Can they see the relevance of your suggestions? As with the practical project, make sure your teacher/lecturer sees this assignment in its draft stages and ensure that you act on any suggestions they make.

GLOSSARY

16PF – Cattell Sixteen Personality Factor Questionnaire: questionniare developed by Cattell (1965) measuring personality in terms of 16 fundamental personality factors

AASQ – Academic Attributional Style Questionnaire: a measure of the explanatory or attributional style used in relation to negative educational events

Acculturative Hassles – problems experienced by people settling in to a new culture/country

ADHD – Attention Deficit Hyperactivity Disorder

Adherence – the extent to which a patient continues the treatment regime agreed with their doctor, for example

African-American Oucher Scale – a scale for measuring pain that uses either numbers or pictures of African-American faces to represent the intensity of pain. It was developed from the Oucher Scale (which used Caucasian faces) specifically for use with African-American children

Ambulatory Blood Pressure – regular, frequent measurement of an individual's blood pressure as they go about their usual daily life

Amsterdamse Biografische Vragenlijst – a personality inventory that measures two dimensions of personality – introversion/extroversion and neuroticism (anxiety)/stability

Angina – (more accurately, angina pectoris) a peculiarly painful disease characterised by a sense of suffocating contraction or tightening of the lower part of the chest

Arthritis Self-Efficacy Scale – a way of measuring the extent to which people with arthritis perceive their ability to function in everyday life

ASVB – Alternative to Suspension for Violent Behaviour: a training programme that includes teaching social problem-solving and thinking skills ... y of reducing violence

...tional style – the characteristic way in which

a person seeks to explain the causes of behaviour

BAI – Beck Anxiety Index: an inventory used to measure anxiety

Barriers to Health Promoting Activities for Disabled Persons Scale – a self-report inventory that measures disabled people's perceptions of what prevents them from taking care of their health

BAS – Body Awareness Scale: a scale measuring self-reported somatic activation experienced by athletes in pre-competitve settings

BAS-II – British Ability Scales (2nd edition) School Age Battery: an intelligence test for school-aged children

B-D HI – Buss-Durkee Hostility Inventory (1975), measuring three types of hostility including assaultive, indirect and verbal

BDI – Beck Depression Inventory: a measure of depression

BEES – Balanced Emotional Empathy Scale: a measure of empathy towards others

Bell Adjustment Inventory – a measure of how well-adjusted a person is in varying situations

Berlin Q-Sort – a 60-item list of statements measuring motivational tendencies

Bloom's Taxonomy – a system that classifies learning into three domains – cognitive, affective, and psychomotor

BMI – Body Mass Index: a measure of body fat based on height and weight

Brigance K&1 Screen – a measure of children's cognitive development

Brown ADD Scales – Brown Attention Deficit Disorder Scales: a test to measure self-perception of attention and organisational skills

CA – communication apprehension: a measure of how willing/unwilling a person is to communicate with others

California Psychological Inventory – an inventory which measures interpersonal behaviour and social interactions

CAP – Child Attention Problems Behaviour Checklist: a measure of attention problems in children

Carotenoids – a class of natural fat-soluble pigments (red, orange and yellow) found principally in plants which, when eaten, serve as antioxidants and a source of vitamin A

CAS – College Alcohol Study: a large scale survey of use of alcohol by American university students conducted by Harvard School of Public Health in 1997, 1999 and 2001

CBA – curriculum-based assessment: an achievement assessment related to the curriculum

CD – Conduct Disorder: a complicated group of behavioural and emotional problems in children characterised by great difficulty in following rules and behaving in a socially acceptable way

CES-D – Centre for Epidemiological Studies Depression Scale: an inventory that measures depression

CHD – coronary heart disease

CIDI-SAM – Composite International Diagnostic Interview Substance Abuse Module: a measure of the extent of substance abuse a person engages in

CIT – Constructive Thinking Inventory: a measure of the degree of constructive/destructive automatic thinking that a person undertakes

Cloninger's TPQ – Cloninger's Tri-dimensional Personality Questionnaire: an inventory that assesses three independent dimensions – novelty seeking (NS), harm avoidance (HA) and reward dependence (RD) – of personality

CNCEQ – Children's Negative Cognitive Error Questionnaire: a measure of distortions in children's thinking

COC – Classroom Observation Code: an observation checklist used to record behaviour in the classroom

Cognitive Tutor – a computer programme used as a teaching aid

COI – Competitive Orientation Inventory: developed by Vealey (1986) and measuring sports confidence

Co-morbidity – a measure of the degree to which two (or more) unrelated conditions occur together

Contingency contract – an agreement between student and teacher that lists behavioural or academic goals and reinforcers or rewards that the student will receive if she/he achieves them

CRIS – Coping Resources Inventory for Stress: a measure of the resources people can call on to help them cope with stress

CSAI-2 – Sports Competition Anxiety Inventory: developed by Martens, Vealey and Burton (1990) and measuring the multidimensional nature of anxiety. Questions relate to cognitive state anxiety, somatic state anxiety and self-confidence

DBD – Disruptive Behaviour Disorder: the collective term given to a number of behavioural disorders including ADHD (Attention Deficit Hyperactivity Disorder), CD (Conduct Disorder) and ODD (Oppositional Defiant Disorder)

Decoding – the skill of extracting the underlying meaning from a written passage

Diabetes Mellitus – a medical condition caused by insufficient production of insulin and resulting in abnormal metabolism of carbohydrates, fats and proteins. There are two types of diabetes mellitus – Type 1 (severe and controlled by injection of insulin) and Type 2 (mild and controlled by diet and exercise)

DISC – Diagnostic Interview Schedule for Children: a measure of conduct disorder

DISC-P – Diagnostic Interview Schedule for Children – Parent Report: a measure of Attention Deficit Hyperactivity Disorder

DSM-III-R – Diagnostic and Statistical Manual of Mental Disorders (3rd edition, revised): the standard diagnostic classification of mental disorders used by mental health professionals in the USA

DUSI – Drug Use Screening Inventory: a measure of the extent of drug misuse

EPQ (or EPI) – Eysenck Personality Questionnaire (or Inventory): a questionnaire that measures personality along the dimensions of Extroversion–Intraversion and Neuroticism–Stability

FABQ – Fear-Avoidance Beliefs Questionnaire: an inventory that measures fear of pain and beliefs about the need to modify behaviour to avoid pain

Faces Pain Rating Scale – a measurement of pain, developed by Wong and Baker, in which children have to select a picture of a face to represent the intensity of pain they are suffering

FBA – functional behavioural analysis: a process of detailed analysis that seeks to identify problem behaviour(s) a student exhibits within an educational environment

Fibromyalgia – a syndrome characterised by chronic pain in the muscles and soft tissues surrounding joints, fatigue, and tenderness at specific sites in the body

Fibromyalgia Impact Questionnaire – a measure of physical, psychological, social and global health

FIRO-B – Fundamental Interpersonal Relations Orientation – Behaviour: a questionnaire measuring interpersonal interactions including inclusion, control and affection

Folate – a type of folic acid

Folic acid – a member of the vitamin B complex group, occurring in green plants, fresh fruit, liver and yeast, and essential for cell growth and reproduction

GCA – General Conceptual Ability

Genotype – the genetic makeup of an organism or virus

GEQ – Group Environment Questionnaire: 18-item questionnaire measuring team cohesion, task cohesion and social cohesion

Gordon Personal Inventory (or Profile) – a Belgian personality inventory based on Cattell's theory of personality

GP – General Practitioner: a doctor that specialises in general health problems – the family doctor

GPA – Grade Point Average: a measure of academic achievement

HAART – Highly Active Anti-Retroviral Therapy: a treatment for HIV/AIDS

Headstart Centre – A centre for the early education of children from disadvantaged backgrounds set up in the USA as part of the Operation Headstart programme

Health Belief Model – a theoretical model that attempts to explain the factors that impact on a person's decisions about whether or not to engage in a health protective behaviour

Homophone – one of two or more words, such as *shear* and *sheer*, that are pronounced the same but differ in meaning, origin and sometimes spelling

Hypertension – abnormally high blood pressure

Hypoglycaemia – lower than normal level of blood glucose

Hypothyroidism – condition resulting from an under-active thyroid gland

IQ – Intelligence Quotient

K-ABC – Kaufman Assessment Battery for Children: an intelligence test for children

K-BIT – Kaufmann Brief Intelligence Test: a standardised intelligence test

LAP – Life Attitude Profile: a measure of the existential meaning and purpose in life (i.e. 'What is life all about?' and 'Why are we here?')

Lateral epicondylitis – tennis elbow: inflammation and pain over the outside of the elbow usually resulting from excessive strain on and twisting of the forearm

LEA – Local Education Authority

Likert scale – a way of measuring attitudes/beliefs by giving a numerical value to the strength of the attitude/belief (e.g. 1 = strongly disagree, 2 = disagree, 3 = neither agree/disagree, 4 = agree, 5 = strongly agree)

Locus of Control – a theoretical construct designed to assess a person's perceived control over his or her own behaviour. Someone with an *internal locus* feels in control of events; whilst someone with an *external locus* perceives others to have that control

LSI – Dunn and Dunn's Learning Style Inventory: a measure of how students prefer to learn

Lynn Achievement Motivation Questionnaire – an eight-item list of self-referent statements measuring achievement motivation

Manual Tender Point Exam – a measurement of pain intensity where patients are asked to rate on a scale of 1–10 the intensity of pain felt when 4kg of pressure is applied consecutively to 18 different sites on the body

McGill Pain Questionnaire – a multi-dimensional inventory used to measure intensity, type, duration and other aspects of pain

MIP – Multisensory Instructional Package: a set of resources which allows the teaching of the same content in a way that maps to different learning styles

MJI – Moral Judgement Inventory: a measure of the stages of moral development and transfer of knowledge

MPQ – Multidimensional Personality Questionnaire: an inventory used to measure a number of different personality dimensions

NARA-II – Neale Analysis of Reading Ability (2nd edition): a test of reading accuracy and comprehension

NCPE – National Curriculum for Physical Education

NTDs – Neural Tube Defects: birth defects occurring in the neural tube, which is the part of the foetus that becomes the spinal cord and brain. The two major types of NTD are anencephaly (the partial or complete absence of the baby's brain) and spina bifida (where vertebrae fail to fuse correctly leaving an opening to the spinal cord)

ODD – Oppositional Defiant Disorder: persistent uncooperative, defiant and hostile behaviour toward authority figures

OLSAT – Otis-Lennon School Ability Test: a cognitive ability test

Oswestry Questionnaire – an inventory for measuring severity of disability

PCS – Perceived Control Scale: a measure of the extent to which people perceive they have control over their day-to-day living

Phoneme – the smallest phonetic unit in a language that is capable of conveying a distinction in meaning, as the *r* of *rate* and the *h* of *hate* in English

Phonological skills – ability to pronounce the sounds of letters/words etc.

Physical Impairment Index – a measure of the degree of impairment resulting from physical injury

PIAT-R – Peabody Individual Achievement Test (Revised)

Pittsburgh Sleep Quality Index – a measure of the quality of sleep a person experiences

POMS – Profile of Mood States: questionnaire developed by McNair, Lorr and Droppleman (1971) measuring a range of mood states including tension, depression, anger, vigour, fatigue and confusion

PPVT-R – Peabody Picture Vocabulary Test – Revised: an achievement test which measures receptive vocabulary – all the spoken words a person can understand

PRCA – Personal Report of Communication Apprehension: a self-report measure of how willing/unwilling a person is to communicate with others

Present Pain Index – a measure of the current intensity of pain

PSS – Perceived Stress Scale: a measure of the extent to which people perceive their life situations and circumstances as stressful

RAN – Rapid Automatized Naming: a test to measure speed and accuracy at naming objects, numbers, letters and letter–number combinations

RAS – Rapid Alternating Stimuli: a test to measure speed and accuracy at naming objects, numbers, letters and letter–number combinations

Raven's Advanced Progressive Matrices – an intelligence test

R-SPQ-2F – the Biggs, Kember, and Leung Two-Factor Revised Study Process Questionnaire: a learning styles inventory which measures how students approach the study of subjects which are important to them

SCAT – Sports Competition Anxiety Test: a questionnaire developed by Martens (1977) measuring competitive trait anxiety

SCS – Self-Control Schedule: a measure of a person's perceptions of the amount of self-control they have over their day-to-day living

Self-efficacy – a person's judgement of his/her own ability to succeed in reaching a goal

Self-Regulating Strategies of Mood – questionnaire measuring strategies used to regulate moods

SENDA – Special Educational Needs and Disabilities Act (2001): an Act of Parliament which places legal requirements on education providers to make all reasonable attempts to accommodate the needs of people with disabilities

SF-36 – Short-Form Health Survey: an inventory that measures general health status

Somatotype – body type or shape

SOQ – Sports Orientation Questionnaire: developed by Gill and Deeter (1988), a 25-item scale measuring three aspects of achievement in sport including competitiveness, win orientation and goal orientation

SPF – sun protection factor: a measure of how much protection against sunburn is given by sunscreen products

Spielberger State Trait Anxiety Inventory – a measure of anxiety in adults

SSQ – Social Support Questionnaire: a measure of the availability of and satisfaction with support from family, friends and neighbours

STAI – State-Trait Anxiety Inventory: developed by Speilberger (1971) and measuring situational state anxiety and general trait anxiety

SWLS – Satisfaction With Life Scale: an inventory that measures how satisfied a person is with their day-to-day life

TAIS – Test of Attentional and Interpersonal Style: a questionnaire developed by Nideffer (1976) including six sub-scales which measure attentional traits

Tinetti Balance Scale – a measure of likelihood of falling

Token economy – a behaviour management technique in which tokens are awarded to students who demonstrate desired behaviours identified by the teacher. Students may periodically exchange the tokens for rewards

VAS – Visual Analogue Scale: an instrument used to measure variables such as pain, e.g. place a mark on the line below to indicate the amount of pain you are currently experiencing:

No pain at all   The worst pain ever

VSQ-9 – Visit Specific Patient Satisfaction Questionnaire: a measure of patient–practitioner relationships

WAIS-R – Wechsler Adult Intelligence Scale (Revised): an intelligence test for adults

WISC-III – Wechsler Intelligence Scale for Children (3rd edition): an intelligence test for children

WOFO – Work and Family Orientation Questionnaire: developed by Helmreich and Spence (1983), this is a general achievement orientation measure with three primary dimensions:
- mastery – the desire for challenge
- work – the desire to work hard
- competitiveness – the desire to win in interpersonal competitions

WRMT-R – Woodcock Reading Mastery Test (Revised): a test of reading ability

WRAT-3 – Wide Range Achievement Test (3rd edition): a test of reading ability

Zuckerman Sensation-Seeking Scale – a measure of the extent to which people seek thrills or play safe